Here's What Others Say About
Dr. Judy's Habit Breakers Stop Smoking Plan:

The Habit Breakers Plan gets down to the basics of quitting smoking. When you complete this Plan, you'll have beaten this habit for good!

--Dick Van Patten, Star of Eight is Enough

The results gained in the Plan are highly encouraging... A well-conceived Plan that works!

--David E. Glass, M.D., Psychiatrist

Smoking is the number one cause of premature labor and small-for-date infants. I recommend the Habit Breakers Plan for any pregnant woman who smokes.

--Randy Harris, M.D., Obstetrician-Gynecologist

Having experienced several stop smoking programs, I found the Habit Breakers approach the most expedient and to the point resulting in a quicker, less painful withdrawal period. The proof is in how I feel—free of smoking and confident of staying free.

--Dave Grusin, Musical Composer, Tootsie and On Golden Pond

T0105504

Dr. Judy's Habit Breakers Stop Smoking Plan

Cold Turkey or Gradual Withdrawal
—With or Without the e-Cigarette

The Choice is Yours

Judy Rosenberg, Ph.D.

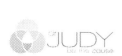

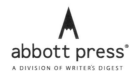

abbott press®
A DIVISION OF WRITER'S DIGEST

Dr. Judy's Habit Breakers Stop Smoking Plan
Cold Turkey or Gradual Withdrawal—With or Without the e-Cigarette

Abbott Press books may be ordered through booksellers or by contacting:

Abbott Press
1663 Liberty Drive
Bloomington, IN 47403
www.abbottpress.com
Phone: 1-866-697-5310

Because of the dynamic nature of the Internet, any web addresses or links contained in this book may have changed since publication and may no longer be valid. The views expressed in this work are solely those of the author and do not necessarily reflect the views of the publisher, and the publisher hereby disclaims any responsibility for them.

Any people depicted in stock imagery provided by Thinkstock are models, and such images are being used for illustrative purposes only.

Certain stock imagery © Thinkstock.

ISBN: 978-1-4582-0493-6 (e)
ISBN: 978-1-4582-0494-3 (sc)

Library of Congress Control Number: 2012912640

Printed in the United States of America

Abbott Press rev. date: 09/06/2012

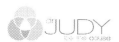

DEDICATION

To my children, Michael, Matthew, and Kineret, their children, and all parents who choose to raise their children to be non-smokers.

Special thanks to my editor, Daniel Linck for his patience and support. With great appreciation.

A special acknowledgement to my deceased father, Leslie Rosenberg for teaching me the basic principles of the Plan, and my mother, Susan Rosenberg, for courageously quitting smoking on her own.

A special THANK YOU to my deceased grandparents Edit and Imre Krausz, for their unconditional love throughout every step of my life.

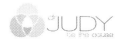

DISCLAIMERS WARNINGS AND RELEASE OF LIABILITY

The information contained in this book is true and complete to the best of our knowledge. The author and publisher disclaim all liability in connection with the use of this information.

WARNING

The rapid-smoking technique contained in this Plan may produce some adverse effects in certain individuals. An alternative technique has been offered for those of you with health conditions or for those of you who are pregnant and may not be able to partake in this part of the Plan. Please check with your doctor or medical practitioner before using this technique.

If you suffer from depression, anxiety, or other mood disorder, you should consult with your doctor or medical practitioner before beginning this Plan.

RELEASE OF LIABILITY

Use the e-Cigarette at your own risk. By using the e-Cigarette in conjunction with the Habit Breakers Stop Smoking Plan you agree to release Dr. Judy Rosenberg and any staff members or individuals connected with this Plan from any and all liability with regard to using the products and techniques recommended, including, but not limited to, the e-Cigarette.

You hereby hold Dr. Rosenberg and Habit Breakers staff members harmless from all product liability claims or other claims regarding your health and participation in the suggested techniques. You understand

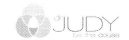

that before engaging in any aspect of the Plan you should consult with your doctor or medical practitioner to insure your safety.

I have read and understood the warning and release of liability regarding all suggested techniques and e-Cigarettes used in conjunction with Dr. Judy's Habit Breakers Stop Smoking Plan.

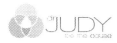

Contents

FOREWORD

As a child, I always pestered my parents to quit smoking, out of concern for my well-being as well as their health. I remember sitting in the back seat of my parent's Chevy, dodging burning ashes from my father's cigarette as they floated toward me. Once, I was burned so badly that I developed a huge blister. It was a tough choice for a child between being burned with the windows open or suffocating from the smoke with the windows closed.

In spite of my dread of cigarettes, I smoked my first when I was 12. I asked my father when I could start smoking. He looked me squarely in the eye and said, "Right now, sweetheart. Let's smoke together." I knew he had something up his sleeve when he lit my first one for me. I smoked my first two cigarettes — it felt like 1/2 a pack. I turned green. I was close to throwing up when he asked me if I'd like another. Needless to say, that was the beginning and the end of my smoking experience.

Smoking a pack-and-a-half a day for over 35 years, my father smoked through two strokes, carotid artery surgery and a coronary triple bypass. He finally quit for a short while after the bypass. It didn't last long — he continued smoking just two days out of intensive care. He actually held a pillow to his chest to ease the pain of coughing while smoking. At age 59 he passed away from pancreatic cancer.

My mother also had problems aggravated by her smoking habit. Smoking a pack a day for 25 years didn't help her damaged heart — she had rheumatic fever as a child. She too underwent open-heart surgery and later required a pacemaker to regulate her heartbeat. She finally quit the habit because she got angry at being controlled by cigarettes. She died of a heart attack at age 67.

If there's one thing I learned from years of pleading with my parents to quit smoking, it's this: You can't talk someone out of smoking. Pleading, bribery, threats and scare tactics don't work. Obviously they haven't worked on you either.

Prior to starting the Habit Breakers Stop Smoking Clinic in 1980, I investigated and worked for many smoking-cessation clinics. I was surprised at what I found. Smokers quitting the habit? Yes. Staying off cigarettes? No. Program participants were relapsing faster than the counselors could treat them — more than half started smoking again within six months. Over 75% of them returned to smoking after one year!

The reasons? Smokers aren't effectively taught to deal with the urge to smoke: They aren't adequately shown how to prevent relapse. They aren't taught how to cope with the emotions that underlie the causes of smoking. And most importantly, they aren't taught how to create a solid support system to help them "stay quit" permanently.

Most programs are more geared to help smokers stop smoking and less to help them stay off. The Habit Breakers Stop Smoking Plan addresses this shortcoming, featuring relapse prevention strategies.

Whenever you are faced with tough emotional issues and your urges to smoke, you will know exactly what to do.

I have created this Plan as an alternative to expensive one-on-one counseling, and to give you the option to quit in the privacy of your own home.

I'm excited to introduce you to two new tools never before used in a smoking cessation plan:

1. The e-Cigarette; and
2. The Mind Map — a Nine Panel model for problem solving, leading you to freedom from your habit and addiction.

You will learn more about these tools in the pages to follow. For those of you who wish to quit smoking without the e-Cigarette as a tool, please know that the Plan can be used with or without it. My intention in creating the Habit Breakers Stop Smoking Plan – Cold Turkey or Gradual Withdrawal/With or Without the e-Cigarette, is to offer you Choice. My ultimate intention is simple: To save or improve the quality of your life.

Wishing You the Best of Health,

Judy Rosenberg, Ph.D

Judy Rosenberg, Ph.D. Founder, Habit Breakers, Inc. (1980).

PREPARING FOR YOUR SUCCESS

COLD TURKEY OR GRADUAL WITHDRAWAL: THE CHOICE IS YOURS

Congratulations on your decision to kick the smoking habit! Whether you choose to quit Cold Turkey, or by Gradual Withdrawal, the Choice Is Yours. If you are a light smoker, if you have experienced stopping smoking and have experienced mild withdrawal symptoms, you may want to opt for Cold Turkey. OR if you simply want to get started and rid your body of nicotine immediately and take the plunge, this may be the way for you to go.

On the other hand, if you are a heavy smoker, have experienced difficulty with nicotine withdrawal in the past, or simply want to take more time to ease off the drug, you may want to opt for Gradual Withdrawal. Either way, the instructions for both Plans are contained in this eBook.

The Plan is divided into Phase 1 (5 days) and Phase 2 (5 days). Phase 1 is the Gradual Withdrawal Phase and Phase 2 is the Cold Turkey Phase.

IF YOU CHOOSE COLD TURKEY: READ DAYS 1 THROUGH 5 AS YOU CONTINUE SMOKING YOUR REGULAR CIGARETTES. YOU MAY COMPLETE THESE SECTIONS SOONER THAN 5 DAYS, BUT DO NOT DRAG OUT YOUR PREPARATION TIME FOR MORE THAN 5 DAYS. CONTINUE TO SMOKE AS MUCH AS YOU LIKE (OR, IF YOU WISH YOU CAN REDUCE YOUR INTAKE AT YOUR LEISURE). AFTER COMPLETING THE READINGS FOR DAYS 1-5, SKIP TO DAY 6, THE DAY YOU GO COLD TURKEY AND BEGIN THE QUIT SMOKING PART OF YOUR STOP SMOKING PLAN.

IF YOU CHOOSE GRADUAL WITHDRAWAL, FOLLOW THE 10 DAY PLAN AS WRITTEN. YOU WILL BE GRADUALLY WEANING OFF NICOTINE FOR 5 DAYS BEFORE YOU GO COLD TURKEY.

WHAT TO EXPECT FROM YOUR PLAN

Thanks to the advent of the e-Cigarette, you will, for the first time in smoking cessation history, have the option to transition from smoking cigarettes to e-Cigarettes, and e-Smoke your way *out* of your habit and addiction.

IMPORTANT CHOICE POINT

I want to make an important statement here: The e-Cigarette is a new tool. Although I have written this Plan to use in conjunction with the e-Cigarette, the Plan was created way before the advent of this tool. You can do the Plan without it. <u>The Choice Is Yours.</u>

If you opt to do the Plan without the e-Cigarette, it's simple: When I refer to the e-Cigarette, use an oral substitute instead, such as a straw or coffee stirrer to fill your oral desire to inhale. If you choose to wean off nicotine using the Gradual Withdrawal Plan without the e-Cigarette, use lower dosage cigarettes instead. Follow the e-Cigarette filter switching schedule by either smoking less or switching to a lower nicotine filtered brand to prepare for Cold Turkey.

If you prefer the Gradual Withdrawal Plan, it is specifically designed to help ease your withdrawal symptoms before you Cold Turkey on nicotine. If you prefer Cold Turkey, you will continue to smoke as usual until Phase 2. Either way, the e-Cigarette or oral substitute is your tool to ease your transition from smoker to ex- smoker, and your Mind Map is your guide to freedom and healing. For your comfort and convenience, your Plan is divided into two phases:

> Phase 1: Five days to prepare your mind and body for success, and wean off the drug nicotine (if you are going Gradual Withdrawal).

Phase 2: Five days to kick the habit permanently and rid your body of nicotine.

This is more than just a how-to-quit-smoking Plan — it's your opportunity to break through your smoking habit and addiction once and for all and lose the desire to resume. During the course of this Plan I refer to cigarettes exclusively, but I also mean any type of nicotine-based tobacco smoked. This step-by-step, gut-level approach consists of a series of exercises designed to eliminate the perceived charm and power of smoking. You will learn to "turn off" your smoking addiction and "turn on" a smoke-free life.

By the time you finish the Habit Breakers Stop Smoking Plan, you will have learned powerful new tools and techniques designed to keep you off cigarettes... permanently!

YOUR FIRST TOOL: YOUR e-CIGARETTE AND e-CIGARETTE SUPPLIES NEEDED

With the advent of the e-Cigarette you can, for the first time in smoking cessation history, make the transition from smoking to nonsmoking easier than ever before. It's the perfect cigarette substitute, and you may be pleasantly surprised to find that by using the e-Cigarette while breaking the habit and addiction, you may not miss smoking as much as you thought you would.

IT'S A "NO BRAINER" SMOKING CESSATION TOOL:

It's not rocket science. Many smokers intuitively find the e-Cigarette to be a successful smoking cessation tool. Here's why:

- The e-Cigarette simulates the pleasure of smoking as it helps you quit the habit.

- If you are doing the Gradual Withdrawal Plan, the e-Cigarette eradicates your craving for nicotine. Like gums and patches, but much more fun and satisfying, it acts as a nicotine delivery system which helps you wean off the drug (Phase 1) before going Cold Turkey.

- The non-nicotine filtered e-Cigarette then transitions you into quitting nicotine altogether (Phase 2).

3

- It's less expensive than gums or patches and you buy it without a prescription.

When you switch from smoking cigarettes to e-Cigarettes, you gain three immediate benefits:

- Say goodbye to tar, carbon monoxide and 4,000 other chemicals, many cancer causing;
- e-Smoke in public if you wish. There is no harmful second hand smoke;
- The e-Cigarette makes quitting easier because it mimics the experience of smoking.

When you switch to your e-Cigarette, say goodbye to:

- Smoking paraphernalia like matches, ashtrays or lighters;
- Bad odor in your mouth, on your hair, clothing, furniture and your whole environment;
- Stained teeth;
- Wasting money on cigarettes — approximately $6 or more if you're a pack-a-day smoker;
- Fire damage;
- Cancer-causing smoke that harms you and others.

Basic e-Cigarette Supplies Needed (available for your convenience at drjudyshabitbreakers.com or at local convenience stores):

COLD TURKEY PLAN:

- E-Cigarette;
- USB charger, wall charger, or car charger, as you prefer;
- Filters   5 or more days supply of zero mg nicotine (flavor only)

GRADUAL WITHDRAWAL PLAN:

- E-Cigarette;
- USB charger, wall charger, or car charger, as you prefer;
- Filters   2 days supply of high (16 mg)

2 days supply of medium (9 mg)

1 day supply of low (6mg)

5 or more days supply of zero mg nicotine (flavor only)

NOTE: If you can't find the exact dosage recommended, use the closest amount of mg's possible to my recommendations. Different companies sell the filters in different dosages and flavors.

Depending on how much you smoke, buy enough supplies to last you through 5 days of Gradual Withdrawal, and 5 days of Cold Turkey. Be sure to buy no more than the amount recommended for the Gradual Withdrawal Phase since you don't want to have extra nicotine filters tempting you beyond the recommended amounts.

FOR EITHER PLAN:

Since smoking zero mg nicotine (flavor only) is harmless, you may want to continue to e-Smoke the zero mg, flavor only filters beyond your Plan, so if you wish, you may want to buy more than a 5 day supply of the flavor only filters. The choice is yours.

After purchasing your supplies, go ahead and familiarize yourself with your e-Cigarette. Learn how to charge it and change the filters. Inhale and see how you like it. On Kick It! Day 1 for Gradual Withdrawal, and Kick It! Day 6 for Cold Turkey, you will substitute your cigarette for your e-Cigarette!

YOUR SECOND TOOL: THE MIND MAP ™

The Mind Map is to help guide you from addiction to healing and freedom.

After years as a practicing clinical psychologist, it occurred to me that client and therapist lacked a simple, effective tool with which to see problems.

Therefore, I created the Mind Map — an effective tool to guide you through three important processes, one for each row of Panels:

FROM the Problem — your addiction,

THROUGH the Process — dismantling your addiction,

TO to the Solution — your pathway to healing and freedom.

The Mind Map is your guide to help you Be The Cause of your success. Notice the three interconnecting circles of my logo. I chose this logo because it represents the transformation you will undergo when you shift from being "at the effect of your addiction and habit" to "being the cause of your freedom and healing."

Stare at the Mind Map on the next page and ask yourself how it might make intuitive sense to you. Note the progression of logic from the 1st Panel, in the upper left, to the 9th Panel, in the lower right, and ask yourself what each Panel might mean.

FROM

THROUGH

TO

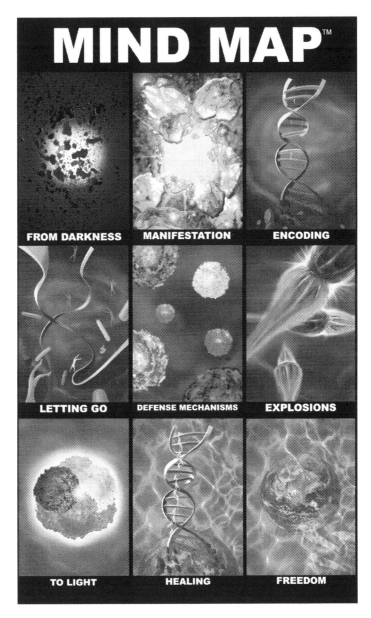

FROM-THROUGH-TO

Okay, now that you've taken your first look at the Mind Map, let's go over each Panel.

Top Row   **FROM — ADDICTION**

PANEL 1 — FROM DARKNESS:

When you first started smoking, you were experimenting. You might have been very young. You had a seemingly valid, yet unenlightened reason for picking up your first cigarette. This could have been an unconscious thought like "I want to look cool," "I want to look grown up," or "I want to rebel," etc. – or just curiosity. Whatever.

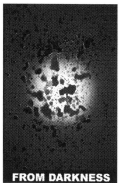

The point is, you were actually coming from an uninformed place — you were in the dark. Panel 1, From Darkness represents this period.

PANEL 2 — MANIFESTATION:

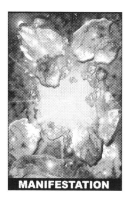

Panel 1's thoughts soon manifested into actual behaviors such as lighting up after a meal, smoking to relieve anxiety, depression or boredom, sharing a social moment with other smokers, etc. The patterns in Panel 1 represent the unique manifestation of your habit.

PANEL 3 – ENCODING:

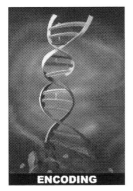

ENCODING

These manifested smoking behaviors, at first innocently experimental and unconscious when you began smoking, quietly started to twist and turn around you like a DNA strand, forming a blueprint of your habit, all the while creating an addiction to nicotine, dictating to you when and how much to smoke. Before you knew it, the blueprint became "encoded" into the fiber of your Being.

THE PRECIPICE

The Precipice is a point of resistance — the point before you take the leap of faith into.....letting go. It's the point at which many smokers consider backing out of their decision to quit smoking. It's a defense against leaving the comfort zone of addiction. Don't be surprised to find yourself ....at the Precipice.

If you are on the Gradual Withdrawal Plan, no worries. The e-Cigarette backs you away from the Precipice to protect you from falling by helping you gradually withdraw from nicotine... easing you towards Cold Turkey. For the first 5 days of your Plan, you will hang out at the Precipice as you wean off nicotine.

If you are on the Cold Turkey Plan, you will have all the psychological tools you need to get past the Precipice to your next phase, Letting Go.

Middle Row   THROUGH — NICOTINE WITHDRAWAL AND STOPPING SMOKING

PANEL 4 – LETTING GO:

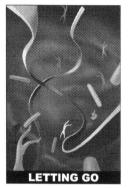

When you finally go Cold Turkey from nicotine (Phase 2, Day 6), the bonds that hold your habit and addiction together break. It's where you really let go and deal with your withdrawal symptoms once and for all.

PANEL 5 – DEFENSE MECHANISMS:

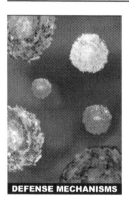

To protect against disorienting feelings associated with nicotine withdrawal, Defense Mechanisms kick in. It's natural for them to appear as you process your feelings of denial, anger, and bargaining with your addiction. These feelings can be masked for only so long before they explode.

PANEL 6 –EXPLOSIONS:

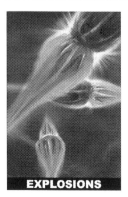

As the Defense Mechanisms break down, your defended feelings are unmasked and expressed as anger, depression, anxiety, etc. During the course of your Plan, you will learn how to deal with these implosions and explosions of feelings without causing injury to yourself or others.

Bottom Row TO — HEALING AND FREEDOM

As you emerge from nicotine withdrawal, a radical change in relating to your habit/addiction occurs. As the dust settles, you will notice a positive shift in your ability to deal with your emotions.

PANEL 7 – TO LIGHT:

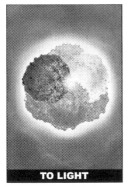

The coming together of your efforts. It's your "A-Ha Moment" — your epiphany — when you recognize your ability to Be The Cause of healing and freeing yourself from addiction.

PANEL 8 — HEALING:

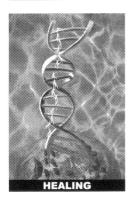

As you heal physically and emotionally, you create a new DNA structure, which becomes the backbone to your newfound health and freedom. Panel 8 represents your healing from Chaos.

PANEL 9 — FREEDOM:

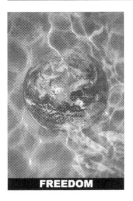

Panel 9 represents the harmony, balance and final integration of your process. The three dolphins represent your hard earned gifts of wisdom, health, and the ability to Be The Cause of your transformation from addiction to freedom.

Print out your Mind Map and take a few minutes to learn it (memorize it). Refer to it often. Post it in a prominent place.

Go to www.drjudyshabitbreakers.com to download a full colored version of your Mind Map.

Your Mind Map will guide you to Be The Cause of your success. It's your Map to freedom.

NO MATTER HOW MUCH OR HOW LONG YOU'VE BEEN SMOKING

Your Plan is designed to help you regardless of how much or how long you've been smoking, and how many times you've tried to quit. Whether it's five cigarettes-a-day or five packs-a-day, whether you've been smoking for one year or 65 years, whether you are quitting for the first time or if you've quit and relapsed many times before, you will learn to deal effectively with all the problems that confront you and learn to find solutions to:

- The chemical and psychological addiction to cigarettes;
- The nagging urge to smoke;
- Relaxing without smoking;
- Controlling your weight;
- Preventing yourself from relapsing;
- Maintaining an on-going support system.

The Habit Breakers Stop Smoking Plan is an active approach to breaking the smoking habit. By participating in a series of exercises designed to turn you off to smoking, you will learn how to break the chain of positive associations you've built up and free yourself from the power of this habit and addiction once and for all!

WHY QUIT SMOKING

SMOKING IS A FREE RIDE THAT CATCHES UP WITH YOU LATER

Perhaps I don't have to tell you that the experience of smoking changes over the lifetime of the addiction. At first, especially during the teenage and young adult years, smoking may seem fashionable, sophisticated, and even sexy.

Because the harmful and painful consequences do not manifest until years later, there is a window of time where it appears that smoking is a free pleasure ride.

Eventually, the pleasure ride catches up. When the price tag of cancer, emphysema, stroke, heart attack and other smoking-related diseases hit on a personal level (over 443,000 smoking related deaths annually), it finally loses all sense of pleasure, sophistication and sex appeal.

By taking a personal inventory of these and other costs of your smoking habit, you build your motivation to quit.

NO MORE SOCIAL TOLERANCE FOR SMOKERS

You've probably noticed a huge change in tolerance towards smokers: Secondhand smoke has become a point of contention for many. Anti-smoking laws prevail — non-smoking restaurant patrons demand to be seated apart from smokers, even in outdoor settings. There's no smoking in movie theatres, airlines and at work. Corporations realize that smoking employees cost them thousands of dollars in increased medical costs, absenteeism, and smoking-related damages, and are happy to go smoke-free.

By now, you've probably experienced the nuisance of leaving a restaurant or theatre for a smoke, fly on an airplane for hours craving nicotine, or worse – get fired from your job for taking too many smoking breaks.

SMOKING IS THE #1 DATING TURNOFF

If you're single and dating, you've probably noticed that unless you're dating a smoker, your habit and addiction is often the cause for being "elimidated." Statistics show that smoking is the #1 dating turnoff. Non-smokers don't want to inhale your secondhand smoke, kiss your smoker's breath, or invest in a partner who has an addiction that can lead to premature disease and death. If you're in a relationship with a non-smoker, chances are you've been nagged about your smoking and its turnoffs.

SMOKING AND PREGNANCY

There is no negotiating on this issue: If you're pregnant and smoking, or if you smoke around your children, STOP IMMEDIATELY!!!

Check out the effects of smoking on your fetus, and the effects of secondhand smoke on your baby or child.

Smoking:

- Lowers the amount of oxygen available to the fetus;

- Increases the heart rate of your fetus;

- Increases your baby's or child's chances of developing respiratory and other health issues;

- Causes your baby or child to develop reduced lung capacity;

- Puts your baby at a higher risk for sudden infant death syndrome (SIDS);

- Is the #1 cause for premature labor and "small-for-date" infants.

More on smoking and pregnancy later.

AN OUTLINE OF YOUR PLAN

IF YOU ARE ON THE COLD TURKEY PLAN:

Your Habit Breakers Cold Turkey Stop Smoking Plan is designed to help you prepare your mind and body for success (Phase 1) before you go Cold Turkey (Phase 2).

The day you quit smoking (Kick It! Day 6) is the day you switch from smoking your cigarettes to smoking your e-Cigarette. Each day you will have a short homework assignment to read to prepare you for your next day. At times you will be asked to write out some homework.

PHASE 1 — PREPARING YOUR MIND AND BODY FOR SUCCESS:

Read chapters 1-5 at your leisure, but take no more than 5 days. Only if you wish, you can reduce your smoking intake, but do not start smoking your e-Cigarette until Phase 2, Day 6, the day you go Cold Turkey.

PHASE 2 — COLD TURKEY:

Five days to break the habit and addiction, and lose the desire to resume. This is the time you switch from smoking cigarettes to smoking your non-nicotine based e-Cigarette filters only. During Phase 2 you will be instructed to "rapid smoke" during the course of the Plan as an aid to help you "turn off" to smoking. The e-Cigarette will continue to be your smoking substitute.

- Day 6-10: Start smoking your zero mg nicotine, flavor only filters.

IF YOU ARE ON THE GRADUAL WITHDRAWAL PLAN:

Your Habit Breakers Gradual Withdrawal Stop Smoking Plan is designed to help you gradually withdraw from nicotine (Phase 1) before you go Cold Turkey (Phase 2).

The day you start your Plan (Kick It! Day 1) is the day you switch from smoking your cigarettes to smoking your e-Cigarette. Each day you will have a short homework assignment to read to prepare you for your next day. At times you will be asked to write out some homework.

PHASE 1 — GRADUAL WITHDRAWAL:

Five days to wean off nicotine.

- Day 1: Switch from smoking cigarettes to smoking your e-Cigarette — High (16 mg) nicotine filter;
- Day 2: Continue to e-Smoke — High (16 mg) nicotine filter;
- Day 3: Switch to Medium (9 mg) nicotine filter;
- Day 4: Continue to e-Smoke — Medium (9 mg) nicotine filter;
- Day 5: Switch to low (6 mg) nicotine filter.

PHASE 2 — GRADUAL WITHDRAWAL — THE COLD TURKEY PART:

Five days to break the habit and addiction, and lose the desire to resume. This is the time you switch from smoking nicotine based e-Cigarettes to smoking non-nicotine based e-Cigarettes only. During Phase 2 you will be instructed to "rapid smoke" during the course of the Plan as an aid to help you "turn off" to smoking. The e-Cigarette will continue to be your smoking substitute.

- Day 6-10: Switch to zero mg nicotine and continue to e-Smoke the flavor only filters.

PREPARING FOR YOUR KICK IT! DAY:

Your Kick It! Day is the day you substitute your cigarette out for your e-Cigarette (Day 6 for Cold Turkey, and Day 1 for Gradual Withdrawal).

On Kick It! Day:

- Refrain from using any nicotine products such as chewing tobacco, pipes, cigars, or Nicotine Replacement Therapy (NRT) like patches or gums;

- Rid your environment of cigarettes, matches, lighters, ashtrays, etc. Make sure to check drawers, pockets, glove compartments, for tobacco and smoking paraphernalia;

- Stop smoking cigarettes and switch to smoking your e-Cigarette;

- Avoid stressful events and alcohol or drug use — they weaken your resolve.

SETTING YOUR HABIT
BREAKERS KICK IT! DATES

You've thought about it, you've talked about it. Perhaps you've made several attempts at it. If you're serious about quitting smoking, there's only one thing left to do — and that's DO IT!

Unless you've recently lost a loved one, or you're in the midst of a divorce or other major life stressors, the best time to quit smoking is NOW! It's a fact of the sabotaging nature of your addiction that the longer you put off your decision to quit, the less likely you ever will. Let's not waste time.

- Pick a comfortable "start" date;
- Schedule your daily sessions around the same time to help your body adjust to nicotine dosage changes;
- Schedule 20 to 40 minutes to complete your daily Plan.

COLD TURKEY:

If you are doing the Cold Turkey Plan, read Days 1-5 at your own leisure, but no more than 5 days to do the reading, and begin your Kick It! Day 6 (the day you go Cold Turkey) as soon as you are ready to Kick It! For Good! You will need 5 consecutive days to complete your Cold Turkey Plan.

PLEASE GET YOUR CALENDAR AND SCHEDULE YOUR 5 CONSECUTIVE DAY PLAN *NOW*.

GRADUAL WITHDRAWAL:

If you are doing the Gradual Withdrawal Plan, you will need 10 consecutive days to complete both Phase 1 (the weaning off phase), and Phase 2 (the Cold Turkey phase).

PLEASE GET YOUR CALENDAR AND SCHEDULE YOUR 10 CONSECUTIVE DAY PLAN *NOW*.

TAKING CARE OF YOURSELF
DURING YOUR PLAN

Turning your Habit Breakers Stop Smoking Plan into a challenging opportunity to create new, more fulfilling ways to relax and reward yourself is completely in your hands. Taking care of yourself is your opportunity to break old unhealthy habits and create a new, healthy lifestyle.

BREAKING THE CHAINS OF YOUR OLD ROUTINES

Imagine getting up bright and early on the morning of your Habit Breakers Kick It! Day (the day you start your Plan), eating a wholesome breakfast, jump-starting your day with exercise, and completing your daily Plan. Imagine comfortably unwinding at the end of the day.

This is your time to break from routine. Go all out! Sleep whenever you need to and can. Buy some flowers or candles and enjoy your newfound sense of smell. Spend a wonderfully relaxing evening at home.

See a movie. Visit friends. Listen to your favorite music. Take up an old hobby or start a new one. Etc...

As you go through the process of quitting smoking, you can either portray yourself as a suffering, frustrated addict in the throes of withdrawal, or as a strong, optimistic individual carving out a new, non-smoking lifestyle. The way you treat yourself will be expressed in how you look, act, and feel, and will influence the way others respond to you.

You can either elicit comments like: "You look like hell," or "You look great! I thought you were quitting smoking this week!"

BREAKING OUT OF YOUR OLD SELF IMAGE

Imagine 10 days filled with massages, facials, manicures, jacuzzis and saunas. It's an ideal time to create a new self image: Join a gym; get a new haircut; shop for new clothes; move some furniture around and change your environment. A "makeover" signals your psyche that you are creating a new, non-smoking lifestyle.

WARNING: STAY WITH YOUR HABIT BREAKERS KICK IT! SCHEDULE.

Do not change your Habit Breakers Stop Smoking Plan dates. Your success is built on your willingness to keep your word to yourself. Your Plan is your top priority.

PHASE 1: GRADUAL WITHDRAWAL OR PREPARING FOR COLD TURKEY

KICK IT! DAY 1: BUILDING MOTIVATION

IF YOU ARE QUITTING COLD TURKEY, PLEASE READ DAYS 1-5 AT YOUR LEISURE, AND CONTINUE SMOKING YOUR CIGARETTES AS USUAL. PLEASE MAKE SURE YOU COMPLETE YOUR READINGS BEFORE DAY 6, THE DAY YOU GO COLD TURKEY. <u>PLEASE IGNORE THE STOP SMOKING CONTRACTS FOR DAYS 1-5.</u>

IF YOU ARE QUITTING GRADUAL WITHDRAWAL, PLEASE BEGIN YOUR PLAN *NOW*: STOP SMOKING YOUR CIGARETTES AND DESTROY ALL REMAINING. START SMOKING YOUR e-CIGARETTE – *BEGIN WITH* HIGH, 16 MG NICOTINE FILTERS.

Reminder:
- Rid your environment of cigarettes, all forms of tobacco and all smoking paraphernalia – matches, lighters, ashtrays, etc.

HOMEWORK: PLEASE READ *NOW*

You may be surprised to learn that most smokers who decide to kick the habit don't do so because they're afraid of dying from a smoking-related disease. Fear of cancer, heart attack, emphysema, stroke, or the many other smoking-related diseases is perceived as something that only happens to the other smoker. Unless it's already happened to you, or you've come to believe that there's immediate danger in continuing to smoke another cigarette, the link between smoking and disease rarely hits home. Most smokers quit for personal reasons.

Some time ago, an 80-year-old man with a history of stroke and high blood pressure came to see me about quitting smoking. He had been smoking a pack a day since he was 13. On the questionnaire beside "How important is it for you to stop smoking?" he answered: "It's urgent that I quit immediately." I asked him why, after 67 years of smoking and living through a stroke did he feel such urgency to quit now? Interestingly, he replied that it wasn't because he was afraid of another stroke. In fact, he told me outright that the idea of dropping dead tomorrow wouldn't bother him at all.

He wanted to quit because his smoker's cough kept him up all night, and he just couldn't bear another night of interrupted sleep. This inconvenience was his motivation to quit.

In a few minutes you will discover your motivation for quitting smoking and use it to reinforce your decision to quit.

There are two basic reasons why you're quitting smoking:

1. The personal consequences you've incurred while smoking.
2. The benefits you expect to attain once you quit.

Perhaps you've had it with the coughing, the lack of energy, or the smell of cigarettes on your body, in your air, or on your clothing and breath. Perhaps you're beginning to feel like a social outcast in a world that's becoming less and less tolerant of smokers. Whatever it is that's personally turning you off to your habit, one thing's certain — the consequences are beginning to, or already have, outweighed the need to continue to smoke.

Perhaps there are certain benefits or payoffs you expect to attain once you've quit. They can be anything from increased physical stamina, a fresher, younger look, saving money, or just a sense of freedom from your reliance on smoking — physically or emotionally.

CHECK OFF THE CONSEQUENCES OF SMOKING AND BENEFITS OF QUITTING

CONSEQUENCES OF SMOKING

1. EMOTIONAL CONSEQUENCES OF SMOKING

- I feel stressed when I smoke.
- I feel depressed after I smoke.
- I don't like using smoking to deal with my frustrations.
- I feel emotionally weak because I smoke.
- I hate giving up my power to a drug.
- I feel nervous and anxious after smoking.
- I hate sneaking around trying to hide my habit.

2. HEALTH CONSEQUENCES OF SMOKING

- Allergies
- Asthma
- Dental problems
- Diabetes
- Emphysema
- Heart attack
- Heart disease
- High blood pressure
- Stroke
- Hyperglycemia

- Ulcer
- Cough
- Sinusitis
- Irritated eyes
- Upset stomach
- Trouble Sleeping
- Pregnancy problems
- Excess sweating
- Heart palpitations
- Chest pains
- Shortness of breath while resting
- Swelling of limbs
- Bad circulation: Cold hands and feet
- Low energy
- Acid stomach and indigestion
- Dull taste and smell
- Trouble with sexual functioning
- Trouble breathing deeply
- Hoarse or husky voice
- Constant mucous in the chest

3.   SOCIAL CONSEQUENCES OF SMOKING

- I'm fed up with being the only one among my friends still smoking.
- I hate feeling like a social outcast.
- I 'm self conscious about my smoker's breath and body odor.
- I've had it with the nagging from friends, family and from my doctor.
- I'm afraid of burning people with cigarettes.
- I'm afraid of losing my job because of smoking breaks.

- My dating life is limited—non-smokers don't date smokers.
- I hate worrying about dirtying up others' environment with my smelly cigarettes.
- I hate polluting the air with my side stream smoke.
- I feel especially guilty smoking around my children.
- I hate being a poor role mode for my children.
- I hate the image I project as a smoker.

4.   IMAGE CONSEQUENCES OF SMOKING

- Embarrassing stains on my teeth.
- My skin looks pale and lifeless.
- My hair looks limp and smells like smoke.
- My hair color is beginning to yellow.
- The crow's feet around my eyes are getting worse.
- The wrinkles between my eyebrows are deeper.
- I'm beginning to see fine lines around my lips – I'm accelerating my aging process.
- My lips are chapped and dry.
- My eyes are bloodshot and irritated.
- My nose is always dripping.
- I look harsh and mean when I smoke.
- My voice is turning harsh and raspy.
- What was once cool, classy, and sophisticated now looks outdated, classless and dirty.

5.   FINANCIAL CONSEQUENCES OF SMOKING

- Cigarettes and other smoking paraphernalia cost a fortune.
- My health insurance premiums are higher.
- I spend a fortune on dry-cleaning bills and laundry.

- I spend more than usual on carpet, drape and upholstery cleaning.
- I'm fed up with repairing holes I've burned in clothes, furniture, and the interior of my car.
- I spend extra on shampoo, cologne, mouthwash, breath mints and smoker's toothpaste.
- I have to get my teeth cleaned more often.
- I lost a potential job because they don't hire smokers.

NOTE: Smoking a pack a day costs over $6.00 a day, and over $2,000 a year. Add on the costs incurred from other financial consequences of smoking and you'll get a more accurate cost of your habit — and the price is only going up!

BENEFITS OF QUITTING

1. EMOTIONAL BENEFITS OF QUITTING

- I'll feel calmer without nicotine in my system.
- I won't feel depressed.
- I'll find more constructive ways of dealing with my frustrations.
- I'll feel powerful conquering my addiction.
- I'll feel empowered to take on other challenges.
- I'll feel emotionally stronger without my crutch.
- I won't have to sneak around other's backs to smoke.
- I'll be treating my body with respect.
- I'll get more done.
- I'll feel proud of accomplishing kicking this habit.

2. HEALTH BENEFITS OF QUITTING

- I will live free of the fear of contracting a smoking related disease.
- My body will have a chance to clean out and recuperate.
- I'll have a healthier pregnancy and baby.
- My smoker's cough will disappear.
- My nasal drip will cease.
- My smoking-related dental problems will disappear.
- Smoking will no longer deplete my body of essential vitamins and minerals.
- I'll have more energy. I'll sleep better.
- No more mucous build-up in my chest.
- My throat won't feel dry and scratchy.
- I won't have problems with indigestion.
- My hoarse voice will clear up. My dental health will be much improved.
- I won't experience morning dizziness from lack of oxygen.
- I won't have to worry about shortness of breath.
- My heart palpitations will go away.
- The swelling in my limbs will go away.
- My circulation will improve and my hands and feet will be warmer.
- I'll be able to breathe deeper and get more oxygen into my system.
- My sexual functioning will improve.
- My sense of taste and smell will improve.
- I'll be calmer without the stimulant nicotine in my body.
- I'll add about 14 years to my lifespan.

3.   IMAGE BENEFITS OF QUITTING

- When I get my teeth cleaned they will stay white.
- My fingers will be clean of yellow stains.
- My tongue won't be coated with tar.
- My skin will look fresher, pinker, and more glowing.
- My bloodshot eyes will look clearer and brighter.
- My hair will smell clean and won't be limp from smoke.
- I won't have nasal drip.
- My clothes will look and smell fresher.
- People will notice my perfume or cologne.
- My makeup, especially my lipstick will stay on longer.
- The lines around my eyes and mouth will soften — I'll prevent premature aging.
- My pockets won't bulge from carrying around cigarettes.
- My face will look friendlier without a cigarette dangling out of my mouth.
- I will convey more strength, energy, success and confidence as an ex-smoker.

4.   FINANCIAL BENEFITS OF QUITTING

- I'll save thousands of dollars a year. My health insurance premiums will decrease.
- I'll save on mouthwash, smoker's toothpaste, cleaning bills, and property damage caused by cigarette burns.
- I'll be more marketable—companies are more likely to hire a non-smoker.

And the MOST important benefit of all:

- My life and health.

Now that you know the reasons why you're quitting smoking, here's how you're going to use them to motivate yourself to get results:

WRITE DOWN YOUR 5 MOST SIGNIFICANT CONSEQUENCES OF SMOKING AND 5 GREATEST BENEFITS OF QUITTING ON POST-IT NOTES, CELL PHONE MEMO PAD, OR WHEREVER YOU POST IMPORTANT NOTES TO YOURSELF. POST THEM ON YOUR BATHROOM MIRROR, NEAR YOUR BED, ON YOUR WORK DESK, AND ON YOUR COMPUTER SCREEN. ETC...DO IT NOW.

SIGN YOUR KICK IT! DAY 1 CONTRACT, AND RETURN TOMORROW AT YOUR SCHEDULED TIME.

PHASE 1: GRADUAL WITHDRAWAL CONTRACT

HABIT BREAKERS GRADUAL WITHDRAWAL

STOP SMOKING CONTRACT FOR KICK IT! DAY 1

I _____, commit to quitting smoking cigarettes permanently. I agree to temporarily transfer my nicotine addiction from cigarettes to my e-Cigarette as I wean off smoking and learn to break the habit and addiction over the course of the 10 Day Plan.

I agree to follow the nicotine dosage schedule below:

- Kick It! Day 1: Switch from smoking cigarettes to smoking your e-Cigarette – High, 16 mg nicotine filter

I understand and agree that I will not "cheat" and smoke cigarettes during the course of Day 1 (or at any other time for that matter), or use nicotine replacement therapy (NRT — gums, patches, or any other form of nicotine, etc.) to supplement my cravings.

I understand that the above dosages are most likely less than I am accustomed to ingesting, and that my withdrawal symptoms will begin as soon as I make the dosage switch from smoking cigarettes to e-Smoking.

I understand that the experience of withdrawal varies from person to person, that they are temporary, and that I can refer to the section on HOW TO HANDLE NICOTINE WITHDRAWAL—Kick It! Day 6, as needed.

I understand that by choosing the Gradual Withdrawal Plan, I am preparing my body to have an easier withdrawal experience when I go Cold Turkey in Phase 2.

I agree to rid my environment of tobacco, cigarettes, matches, lighters, ashtrays, and other smoking paraphernalia.

I am quitting smoking for myself, and of my own free will and I'm choosing to do so for the following reasons:

MY 5 MOST IMPORTANT BENEFITS OF QUITTING:

1. _____

2. _____

3. _____

4. _____

5. _____

Signed _____

Dated _____

PHASE 1: GRADUAL WITHDRAWAL OR PREPARING FOR COLD TURKEY

KICK IT! DAY 2: DEVELOPING AN ATTITUDE FOR SUCCESS

FOR GRADUAL WITHDRAWAL ONLY: PLEASE CONTINUE SMOKING YOUR e-CIGARETTE – HIGH, 16 MG NICOTINE FILTER

Reminder:
- Rid your environment of cigarettes, all forms of tobacco and all smoking paraphernalia — matches, lighters, ashtrays, etc.

HOMEWORK: PLEASE READ *NOW*

Inside each and every smoker, and you are no exception, is a part I call the addict. The addict is that part of you that wants to walk away and forget about quitting smoking. It says, "I'll do It later." It's the part that believes that without cigarettes, you'll get fat... or be unable to cope with your job, your family, or the stress of life. The part that believes you need cigarettes to survive, no matter what the consequences to your health.

Since the moment you decided to take action, your addict has been devising intricate excuses why you can't or shouldn't quit. The addict needs these Defense Mechanisms to protect you from the terrible consequences you believe will result from quitting smoking.

Although logically you know that you won't fall apart without smoking, your addict doesn't believe it and will try anything to sabotage your attempt. Really, anything.

Fortunately, you can learn to use your addict to work for, rather than against you. In the following exercise you will learn how it thinks and behaves, and how it tries to get you to give up the idea of quitting. By learning how to respond to your addict, you can learn to beat it at its own game.

ADDICT THOUGHTS AND BEHAVIORS

FROM BE THE CAUSE TO *BECAUSE*:

Your addict is the part of you that wants to sabotage your attempts at stopping smoking by devising a mountain of excuses to get you to give up the idea of quitting smoking. It wants to take away your power to Be The Cause of your success and leave you with excuses why. "I can't because..." Here are some common excuses smokers use to avoid quitting, and how you can respond to them:

Addict: "If I quit smoking, I'll get fat. I'd rather be a thin smoker than a fat ex-smoker."

Self-Talk: "Who am I kidding? There are plenty of smokers who quit the habit and regulate their weight, just as there are plenty of overweight smokers. Smoking is not the answer to weight control. If I put on some excess pounds, I'll do something about it instead of using it as an excuse to go back to smoking."

Addict: "I've been smoking for too many years. I've tried to quit many times, and can't even make it through the first half of my day without a cigarette. It feels hopeless, so why bother trying?"

Self-Talk: "Why bother? Because I don't really believe it's hopeless. Millions of smokers have kicked the habit, some, heavier smokers than I. This time I have the Plan and the e-Cigarette, and Mind Map to help me through."

Addict: "I can't relax without a cigarette. It's my reward. It's my last and only vice.

Self-Talk: "What kind of a reward is a 'cancer stick'?"

Addict: "Cigarettes make me feel more comfortable socially. I'll feel awkward if I don't have my security blanket beside me."

Self-Talk: "I want to stop hiding behind cigarettes and meet new people."

Addict: "I won't be able to deal with stress without cigarettes."

Self-Talk: "For years I've been shoving down my unpleasant feelings by smoking. This method of relieving tension is causing more problems than it's relieving. I'll find healthier ways to cope."

Addict: "Smoking's not so bad for you. My grandfather smoked two packs a day for over 70 years and he's still going strong at age 90."

Self-Talk: "My grandfather's lucky. Who knows if I'll be lucky too. There is no denying that smoking is a deadly habit, and I'm not willing to take any chances with my life and health."

PLEASE FILL OUT. WRITE DOWN YOUR ADDICT
VERSES SELF TALK CONVERSATIONS

Addict_____

Self-Talk_____

Addict_____

Self-Talk_____

Addict_____

Self-Talk_____

Addict_____

Self-Talk_____

The e-Cigarette has been created to transition you out of your habit and nicotine addiction. With this unique tool, never has there been a better time to kick the habit!

You may find that your sabotaging thoughts may gain strength to the point that you may be tempted to cancel your "Kick It! Day," such as:

- "I remember I have an important business deal to complete;"
- "I remember that my uncle is coming to visit and I can't entertain and quit smoking at the same time;"
- "Perhaps I'll run myself down, catch a cold or the flu." Etc.

You'd be amazed how the mind and body work together to sabotage quitting.

Remember, you're at "The Precipice" — the period before you go Cold Turkey. The Precipice is where many smokers get "cold feet" and want to back away.

I'm not suggesting that there couldn't be valid reasons at present that warrant postponing your Plan. For instance... quitting smoking if you are currently under unbearably stressful circumstances, such as divorce, job loss, a death in the family, etc. What I am suggesting is that life is full of ups and downs, and there will always be reasons why quitting now is "out of the question." Prioritize how important your quitting smoking is to you and act.

If you hear yourself give excuses like "Not today, I have to shampoo the dog," or "Not now, my horoscope advises against it," etc., you can bet that your addict is at work.

PLEASE FILL OUT. WRITE DOWN 3 EXCUSES WHY NOT TO QUIT AND THE COUNTERACTING SELF-TALK.

Excuse:_____

Self-Talk:_____

Excuse_____

Self-Talk_____

Excuse_____

Self-Talk_____

FOR GRADUAL WITHDRAWAL ONLY: PLEASE SIGN YOUR KICK IT! DAY 2 CONTRACT AND RETURN TOMORROW AT YOUR SCHEDULED TIME.

PHASE 1: GRADUAL WITHDRAWAL CONTRACT

HABIT BREAKERS GRADUAL WITHDRAWAL

STOP SMOKING CONTRACT FOR KICK IT! DAY 2

I _____, commit to quitting smoking cigarettes permanently. I agree to temporarily transfer my nicotine addiction from cigarettes to my e-Cigarette as I wean off smoking and learn to break the habit and addiction over the course of the 10 Day Plan.

I agree to follow the nicotine dosage schedule below:

- Kick It! Day 2: Continue smoking your e-Cigarette – High, 16 mg nicotine filter

I understand and agree that I will not "cheat" and smoke cigarettes during the course of Day 2 (or at any other time for that matter), or use nicotine replacement therapy (NRT — gums, patches, or any other form of nicotine, etc.) to supplement my cravings.

I understand that the above dosages are most likely less than I am accustomed to ingesting, and that my withdrawal symptoms began as soon as I made the dosage switch from smoking cigarettes to e-Smoking.

I understand that the experience of withdrawal varies from person to person, that they are temporary, and that I can refer to the section on HOW TO HANDLE NICOTINE WITHDRAWAL—Kick It! Day 6, as needed.

I understand that by choosing the Gradual Withdrawal Plan, I am preparing my body to have an easier withdrawal experience when I go Cold Turkey in Phase 2.

I agree to rid my environment of tobacco, cigarettes, matches, lighters, ashtrays, and other smoking paraphernalia.

I am quitting smoking for myself, and of my own free will and I'm choosing to do so for the following reasons:

MY 5 MOST IMPORTANT BENEFITS OF QUITTING:

1. _____

2. _____

3. _____

4. _____

5. _____

Signed _____

Dated _____

PHASE 1: GRADUAL WITHDRAWAL OR PREPARING FOR COLD TURKEY

KICK IT! DAY 3: PREPARING TO GO COLD TURKEY

FOR GRADUAL WITHDRAWAL ONLY: PLEASE SWITCH TO SMOKING YOUR e-CIGARETTE — MEDIUM, 9 MG NICOTINE FILTER

Reminder:
- Rid your environment of cigarettes, all forms of tobacco and all smoking paraphernalia — matches, lighters, ashtrays, etc.

HOMEWORK: PLEASE READ *NOW*

EATING RIGHT

While your body is detoxifying, pay attention to your diet. This is a good time to eat the freshest and healthiest foods possible. Organic is always best.

Some Common Sense Rules:

It's a great time to become a "label-reader:"

- Reduce significantly the amounts of preservatives, trans fats and artificial chemicals;

- Minimize your salt intake to avoid water retention;

- Minimize your sugar intake to avoid empty calories;

- Drink plenty of water to flush out nicotine and other toxins stored in your body.

(NOTE: When drinking plain ("tap"), mineral, or carbonated water, make sure it's low sodium to prevent water retention. Distilled water is best.)

FOODS TO CHOOSE

To help keep your energy level consistent while withdrawing from nicotine, choose from the following food groups:

Fresh fruits and vegetables (preferably organic, at least 5-6 servings/day);

Dairy products (organic low fat milk, cheeses, butter, Greek yogurt, etc.) (2-3 servings/day);

Whole-grain breads and cereals (again, organic — sprouted or flourless breads, oatmeal, etc. Shy away from sugar-coated or fatty rolls such as Danish or cinnamon rolls, pastries, cake, croissants, etc.) (3-4 servings/day);

Proteins, such as organic nuts (walnuts, almonds, etc.), legumes (beans, chick peas, hummus, soy, tofu, etc.), whole eggs and lean meats (turkey, fish, chicken) (3-5 servings/day).

NOTE: Smokers (and all those exposed to second-hand smoke) should consume more foods high in:

- Beta-carotene (carrots, squash, yams, sweet potatoes and other yellow-orange vegetables such as peppers);
- Vitamin C (citrus fruits, broccoli, bell pepper) and;
- Vitamin E (wheat germ, nuts).

FOODS TO AVOID

To avoid triggering nicotine cravings, avoid:

- Sugar
- Carbonated beverages
- White flour
- Red meat
- Alcohol
- Coffee

SHOPPING BEFORE YOU QUIT

Before Habit Breakers Kick It, Day 6, the day you go Cold Turkey, I suggest that you pick up a few items to boost your health as you quit.

DETOXIFYING and ANTI-INFLAMMATORY TEAS:

- Calming: Anise, Valerian, Chamomile
- Soothing for the Lungs: Elecampane, Ginseng
- Antioxidant: Green Tea, Pomegranate
- Anti-Inflammatory: Ginger

SUGAR SUBSTITUTES:

- Stevia or Truvia — zero calorie herbal sugar substitutes made from plant extract;
- Agave — a plant based nectar that saves calories and has a low glycemic index.

Stay away from artificial sweeteners such as aspartame, Splenda, Equal Sweet n' Low and NutraSweet. These sweeteners are neurotoxins and are responsible for hundreds of negative symptoms.

ORGANIC FRUITS AND VEGETABLES:

- Carrots, beets, squash, yams, sweet potatoes — vitamin rich;
- Apples, berries, watermelon— high in antioxidants; helps flush out toxins and fight disease;
- Lemons, oranges, grapefruit – high in Vitamin C to counteract the damages of smoking;
- Bok Choy — best anti-inflammatory vegetable — cook or great in salads.

Try juicing your fruits and vegetables for easier absorption to cleanse your system.

DAIRY FOR ADDED CALCIUM:

- Milk, Buttermilk, Kefir, Yogurt, Cottage Cheese.

HIGH FIBER, FOR VITAMINS AND MINERALS: VEGETABLES AND LEGUMES

- Broccoli, cauliflower, carrots, spinach, green beans, kale, beets, chick peas (garbanzos), kidney beans, artichokes, peppers — the fresher the better — try to find organic or locally-grown. Non-frozen.

WHOLE GRAINS

- Whole grain breads and cereals — oats, barley, quinoa, wheat germ, brown rice – keeps your bowels moving;
- Black rice — a spoonful contains anthocyanin, a very helpful antioxidant.

PROTEINS TO SUSTAIN ENERGY AND REPAIR TISSUE:

- Fish — wild-caught if possible (remember there is a high mercury content currently in most fish, especially tuna)
- Chicken — organic, kosher, antibiotic and hormone-free
- Soy products — tofu, edamame, soy milk, etc.
- Eggs — hard-boiled, poached, anything but fried
- Beans — garbanzos, kidney, black, etc.
- Nuts and Seeds — walnuts, almonds, flax, soy, etc.

GOOD FATS

- Avocados
- Flax seed, sesame, and olive oil
- Nuts – walnuts, almonds, cashews, etc.
- Fatty fish — salmon, tilapia, sea bass

Good fats increase "good" cholesterol (HDL), and lower "bad" cholesterol (LDL).

BAD FATS

- Butter (ok in moderation)
- Fatty meats
- Fried foods

TRANS FATS

Read labels and beware of Trans Fats found in:
- Butter-like spreads (margarines)
- Packaged and canned foods (especially soups)
- Fried foods
- Frozen foods

Trans Fats raise your LDL (bad) cholesterol increasing your risk of stroke and heart disease.

CIGARETTE SUBSTITUTES

Although the e-Cigarette is your primary cigarette substitute, here are some alternatives to fill the void of smoking:

ORAL SUBSTITUTES

As you withdraw from smoking, you may feel the need to replace the oral gratification once satisfied by your cigarette. Like habitual muscle memory, the feeling of the cigarette in your mouth provided a kind of comfort. You will most likely feel tempted to fill this void with food, gum and other substances that involve use of the mouth, tongue, taste, muscle movements and other subliminal oral involvement.

To avoid putting the wrong substances (fattening foods, tobacco, etc.) in your mouth, choose from the following:

HEALTHY SNACKS

- Fruits and vegetables (cut into bite-sized pieces)
- Non-fat popcorn

- Rice cakes
- Whole wheat crackers
- Sunflower seeds
- Be mindful of quantity — over-eating even low calorie snacks can cause weight gain.

NON-FOOD ORAL SUBSTITUTES

Non-food oral substitutes are the best prevention against compulsive eating giving the mouth muscles and tissues "something to do" now that your cigarette habit is being replaced. Choose from the following:

- Cinnamon sticks
- Coffee stirrers
- Straws
- Toothpicks (try some from health food stores which have tea tree oil and cinnamon)
- Sugar free gum
- Sugar free mints

TACTILE SUBSTITUTES

Your fingers, hands and arms, (and all supporting muscles and nerves) used for movements associated with your cigarette (lighting, raising to take a drag, flicking ash, pounding out in a tray, etc.) will now feel something missing as well. Consider the following tactile substitutes:

- Pencil or pen (try doodling)
- Cell phones - games, texting, email, photos, etc.
- Small hand gaming devices
- Beads
- Smooth stones
- Grip exercisers
- Play dough or modeling clay

VITAMINS AND MINERALS

To begin healing your body from the damage of your prior smoking, supplement your diet with a multivitamin and mineral plan for at least one month after quitting...and keep it as part of your daily regimen.

According to Dr. Ronald Thompson, the former director of Vitamin and Supplement Research and Development of General Nutrition Inc., the body's need for vitamins and minerals are increased after you stop smoking. Make sure your vitamin supplements contain:

- Vitamin E — (200 mg) antioxidant that helps prevent heart disease and stroke-causing scars on arterial walls;
- Vitamin C — (1000 mg) eases stress, replenishes supply robbed by smoking;
- Vitamin B1— (thiamine) calming effects;
- Vitamin B5 — (pantothenic acid) calming effects;
- Vitamin B6 — (pyridoxine) diuretic to help with water retention;
- Selenium — acts to prevent toxic deposits of heavy metals like cadmium;
- Magnesium — body stress from smoking toxins causes magnesium levels to fall, affecting cholesterol levels.

FOR GRADUAL WITHDRAWAL ONLY: PLEASE SIGN YOUR KICK IT! DAY 3 CONTRACT AND RETURN TOMORROW AT YOUR SCHEDULED TIME.

PHASE 1: GRADUAL WITHDRAWAL CONTRACT

HABIT BREAKERS GRADUAL WITHDRAWAL

STOP SMOKING CONTRACT FOR KICK IT! DAY 3

I _____, commit to quitting smoking cigarettes permanently. I agree to temporarily transfer my nicotine addiction from cigarettes to my e-Cigarette as I wean off smoking and learn to break the habit and addiction over the course of the 10 Day Plan.

I agree to follow the nicotine dosage schedule below:

- Kick It! Day 3: Switch to smoking your e-Cigarette – Medium, 9 mg nicotine filter

I understand and agree that I will not "cheat" and smoke cigarettes during the course of Day 3 (or at any other time for that matter), or use nicotine replacement therapy (NRT — gums, patches, or any other form of nicotine, etc.) to supplement my cravings.

I understand that the above dosages are most likely less than I am accustomed to ingesting, and that my withdrawal symptoms began as soon as I made the dosage switch from smoking cigarettes to e-Smoking.

I understand that the experience of withdrawal varies from person to person, that they are temporary, and that I can refer to the section on HOW TO HANDLE NICOTINE WITHDRAWAL—Kick It! Day 6, as needed.

I understand that by choosing the Gradual Withdrawal Plan, I am preparing my body to have an easier withdrawal experience when I go Cold Turkey in Phase 2.

I agree to rid my environment of tobacco, cigarettes, matches, lighters, ashtrays, and other smoking paraphernalia.

I am quitting smoking for myself, and of my own free will and I'm choosing to do so for the following reasons:

MY 5 MOST IMPORTANT BENEFITS OF QUITTING:

1. _____

2. _____

3. _____

4. _____

5. _____

Signed _____

Dated _____

PHASE 1: GRADUAL WITHDRAWAL OR PREPARING FOR COLD TURKEY

KICK IT! DAY 4: SETTING UP A SUPPORT SYSTEM

FOR GRADUAL WITHDRAWAL ONLY: PLEASE CONTINUE TO SMOKING YOUR e-CIGARETTE – MEDIUM, 9 MG NICOTINE FILTER

Reminder:

- Rid your environment of cigarettes, all forms of tobacco and all smoking paraphernalia — matches, lighters, ashtrays, etc.

HOMEWORK: PLEASE READ *NOW*

Getting support while you quit smoking can make a big difference to your morale and success. Here are 3 options for setting up a support system:

1. Enlist the support of your spouse, significant other, friend, or family member. Ask them to listen if and when you need to vent;

2. Quit smoking with a buddy, but only if he or she is as serious about quitting smoking as you are. Make plans to see a movie, exercise, dine out, or just spend a quiet evening together. Make an agreement that, before lighting up a cigarette, you will call each other for support.

3. Try attending free support groups in your community, such as Smoker's Anonymous.

Informing friends, family, and significant others about the start-date of your Plan makes your commitment public and gives you added incentive to stay with your **Habit Breakers** *Kick It! Date*.

Ask those around you — at home, at work, etc. — to be patient and supportive as you adjust to the chemical and psychological changes associated with nicotine withdrawal and breaking your smoking habit. **Let your needs be known.**

24-HOUR CRISIS INTERVENTION STOP SMOKING HOTLINE

Research has shown that the most effective smoking cessation plan is one that provides ongoing support. Set up your own 24-Hour Crisis Intervention Hotline with someone willing to be on call for you – even for a short while — who can offer support if you are feeling the urge to light up.

FOR GRADUAL WITHDRAWAL ONLY: PLEASE SIGN YOUR KICK IT! DAY 4 CONTRACT AND RETURN TOMORROW AT YOUR SCHEDULED TIME.

PHASE 1: GRADUAL WITHDRAWAL CONTRACT

HABIT BREAKERS GRADUAL WITHDRAWAL

STOP SMOKING CONTRACT FOR KICK IT! DAY 4

I _____, commit to quitting smoking cigarettes permanently. I agree to temporarily transfer my nicotine addiction from cigarettes to my e-Cigarette as I wean off smoking and learn to break the habit and addiction over the course of the 10 Day Plan.

I agree to follow the nicotine dosage schedule below:

* Kick It! Day 4: Continue smoking your e-Cigarette – Medium, 9 mg nicotine filter

I understand and agree that I will not "cheat" and smoke cigarettes during the course of Day 4 (or at any other time for that matter), or use nicotine replacement therapy (NRT — gums, patches, or any other form of nicotine, etc.) to supplement my cravings.

I understand that the above dosages are most likely less than I am accustomed to ingesting, and that my withdrawal symptoms began as soon as I made the dosage switch from smoking cigarettes to e-Smoking.

I understand that the experience of withdrawal varies from person to person, that they are temporary, and that I can refer to the section on HOW TO HANDLE NICOTINE WITHDRAWAL—Kick It! Day 6, as needed.

I understand that by choosing the Gradual Withdrawal Plan, I am preparing my body to have an easier withdrawal experience when I go Cold Turkey in Phase 2.

I agree to rid my environment of tobacco, cigarettes, matches, lighters, ashtrays, and other smoking paraphernalia.

I am quitting smoking for myself, and of my own free will and I'm choosing to do so for the following reasons:

MY 5 MOST IMPORTANT BENEFITS OF QUITTING:

1. _____

2. _____

3. _____

4. _____

5. _____

Signed _____

Dated _____

PHASE 1: GRADUAL WITHDRAWAL OR PREPARING FOR COLD TURKEY

KICK IT! DAY 5: A LAST WORD BEFORE YOU GO COLD TURKEY

FOR GRADUAL WITHDRAWAL ONLY: PLEASE SWITCH TO SMOKING YOUR e-CIGARETTE – LOW, 6 MG NICOTINE

Reminder:

- Rid your environment of cigarettes, all forms of tobacco and all smoking paraphernalia — matches, lighters, ashtrays, etc.

HOMEWORK: PLEASE READ *NOW*

AMBIGUITY: TRYING DOESN'T WORK

"Giving up smoking is the easiest thing in the world. I know because I've done it thousands of times" — Mark Twain

Quitting smoking and quitting smoking *permanently* are two different concepts. Any smoker, including you, can give up smoking... temporarily. So what's the secret to quitting permanently?

After years of working with thousands of smokers I can tell you what doesn't work: Trying to quit.

Trying is an ambiguous lie you create to sabotage your success — it's a recipe for failure. Trying implies that you might not succeed, creating hope to smoke in the future. It's your loophole out.

CLOSING THE CIRCLE OF AMBIGUITY

BE THE CAUSE

Look at your Mind Map, Panel 1 — From Darkness. As you read the following, notice the dark and light areas in the Panel. The dark areas represent your addiction. The light areas represent the source of your power to be successful.

Your addiction loves ambiguity. If you give your addict mind a loophole to escape, it will. A 99% commitment creates a 1% escape hatch— just enough to re addict yourself. That is why nothing short of a 100% commitment works.

Closing the circle of ambiguity takes you out of Darkness (addict thinking) and activates your Light – your power to Be the Cause of your success. By substituting trying with committing, and by making a 100% commitment to quitting smoking, you close the circle and set your intention to succeed.

You've just learned "the secret" to success: A 100 % Commitment — it's the source of your power.

You're now familiar with the sabotaging nature of your addiction; you're almost nicotine-free; you've learned to cope with the thoughts and behaviors that impede success. You are mentally and physically prepared, and you have the e-Cigarette and Mind Map to transition and guide you through.

"Activate your Light" now — COMMIT IN WRITING to go Cold Turkey.

FOR GRADUAL WITHDRAWAL ONLY: PLEASE SIGN YOUR KICK IT! DAY 5 CONTRACT AND RETURN TOMORROW AT YOUR SCHEDULED TIME.

PHASE 1: GRADUAL WITHDRAWAL CONTRACT

HABIT BREAKERS GRADUAL WITHDRAWAL

STOP SMOKING CONTRACT FOR KICK IT! DAY 5

I _____, that today is the last day that I will be smoking nicotine based e-Cigarette filters, and that tomorrow I will be going Cold Turkey on nicotine. I agree to temporarily transfer my nicotine addiction from cigarettes to my e-Cigarette as I wean off smoking and learn to break the habit and addiction over the course of the 10 Day Plan.

I agree to follow the nicotine dosage schedule below:

- Kick It! Day 5: Switch to smoking your e-Cigarette – Low, 6 mg nicotine filter

I understand and agree that I will not "cheat" and smoke cigarettes during the course of Day 5 (or at any other time for that matter), or use nicotine replacement therapy (NRT — gums, patches, or any other form of nicotine, etc.) to supplement my cravings.

I understand that the above dosages are most likely less than I am accustomed to ingesting, and that my withdrawal symptoms began as soon as I made the dosage switch from smoking cigarettes to e-Smoking.

I understand that the experience of withdrawal varies from person to person, that they are temporary, and that I can refer to the section on HOW TO HANDLE NICOTINE WITHDRAWAL—Kick It! Day 6, as needed.

I understand that by choosing the Gradual Withdrawal Plan, I am preparing my body to have an easier withdrawal experience when I go Cold Turkey tomorrow in Phase 2.

I agree to rid my environment of tobacco, cigarettes, matches, lighters, ashtrays, and other smoking paraphernalia.

I am quitting smoking for myself, and of my own free will and I'm choosing to do so for the following reasons:

MY 5 MOST IMPORTANT BENEFITS OF QUITTING:

1. _____

2. _____

3. _____

4. _____

5. _____

Signed _____

Dated _____

You just "activated your Light" and took the most significant step in Being The Cause of your success — COMMITING to going COLD TURKEY!

CONGRATULATIONS!

YOU HAVE JUST COMPLETED
PHASE 1:
ONTO
PHASE 2: COLD TURKEY!

SUPPLIES NEEDED FOR TOMORROW:

1 PACK OF YOUR REGULAR CIGARETTES

(PURCHASE THEM BEFORE TOMORROW'S SESSION)

LIGHTER OR MATCHES

LARGE GLASS JAR WITH A LITTLE WATER

(FOR DISCARDING YOUR BUTTS)

<u>WARNING</u>: DO NOT OPEN YOUR PACK OF CIGARETTES UNTIL YOU ARE INSTRUCTED TO DO SO IN TOMORROW'S SESSION WHEN YOU WILL BE INSTRUCTED TO SMOKE "TUR OFF STYLE" !!!! IT IS VITAL TO THE SUCCESS OF YOUR PLAN THAT YOU FOLLOW ALL INSTRUCTIONS. YOU MAY SMOKE YOUR e-CIGARETTE BETWEEN SESSIONS. IT'S YOUR CIGARETTE SUBSTITUTE!

PHASE 2: COLD TURKEY

KICK IT! DAY 6: NICOTINE WITHDRAWAL/ TURNING OFF TO SMOKING

PLEASE SWITCH TO SMOKING YOUR e-CIGARETTE – ZERO MG NICOTINE FILTER, FLAVOR ONLY

Reminder:

- Rid your environment of cigarettes, all forms of tobacco and all smoking paraphernalia — matches, lighters, ashtrays, etc.

HOMEWORK: PLEASE READ *NOW*

Important: <u>Don't open your pack of cigarettes until you are instructed to smoke</u>. It's vital to the success of the program that you wait for instructions.

Welcome to Phase 2: Cold Turkey. If you spent the last 5 days weaning off nicotine, you've made great progress ridding your system of the drug and decreasing the time line and intensity of your withdrawal symptoms. If you are on the Cold Turkey Plan, no worries. Your body will naturally rid itself of nicotine within approximately 48 to 72 hours (depending on how much you smoke).

Congratulations!

You are now entering the middle row of your Mind Map: THROUGH WITHDRAWAL AND STOPPING SMOKING. You will be traveling THROUGH this phase for the next few days while you detox from nicotine and learn to break your smoking habit. It's your most challenging phase and I ask that you be patient and kind to yourself as you journey THROUGH.

IMPORTANT NOTE: PEASE HAVE YOUR PACK OF CIGARETTES, LIGHER OR MATCHES AND YOUR LARGE GLASS JAR FILLED WITH WATER READY. TODAY YOU WILL BE INSTRUCTED TO RAPID-SMOKE "TURN OFF" STYLE. UNTIL THEN, DO NOT OPEN YOUR PACK OF CIGARETTES!

According to former Surgeon General C. Everett Koop, nicotine is one the most addicting drug known to man; as addicting as heroin and cocaine. Nicotine is so powerful that it tricks the brain into abandoning life enhancing survival mechanisms in favor of obtaining the drug. That is why so many smokers, over 443,000 deaths per year in the United States alone, die of a smoking-related illness. Not even serious health consequences or threat of dying can get in the way of the drug. A case in point — during World War II Jews starving for food during the time of holocaust would sometimes trade food for cigarettes. So powerful is the drug.

UNDERSTANDING NICOTINE ADDICTION

Why is it so difficult to stop smoking?

According to the Nicotine Addiction Model, smokers smoke to avoid experiencing nicotine withdrawal (listed in the next section).

Every 20 minutes or so, the level of nicotine in your system drops, triggering your urge to smoke. What's interesting is that the pleasure, or "euphoria" of smoking is experienced before the drug hits the brain, not after the nicotine craving is satisfied. In other words, the pleasure is sensed before your brain registers the "nicotine hit."

The pleasure you derive from smoking has more to do with inhaling deeply and is merely incidental to fulfilling your body's need for the drug. Inhaling your e-Cigarette delivers immediate pleasure, even though it contains no nicotine. It's your perfect cigarette substitute!

Except for the first cigarette of the day, which functions mostly to satisfy your need for nicotine, much of your smoking is prompted by internal and external cues or "triggers" (stress, eating, drinking coffee, etc.). To support this notion, research shows that craving for nicotine plays a less prominent role in relapse — 90% of smokers have a behavioral dependence verses a chemical addiction. Only 21% experience severe nicotine withdrawal.

Statistically, you're already ahead of the game because you've spent five days weaning off the drug. So let's continue.

THE PHYSIOLOGICAL EFFECTS OF NICOTINE ON THE BRAIN

Let's look at nicotine's effect on your brain to understand why it's so addicting:

FREE BASE NICOTINE — WOW, WHAT A HOOK!

In general, tobacco companies are very savvy about maintaining high profits by highly unethical ways of hooking you and keeping you stuck. They've changed the chemical property of nicotine by adding ammonia, essentially creating a "free-base version" of nicotine — much more potent and addicting than regular nicotine! When you smoke this "free-base nicotine," the effects are super-addicting!

Feel manipulated?

The tobacco companies obviously know how to encode the addiction into the fiber of your Being and essentially keep you enslaved for life. (Have they been studying the Mind Map, Panel 3 — Encoding?)

HOW TO HANDLE NICOTINE WITHDRAWAL

By the time you complete this section, you will know how to handle your cravings for nicotine. In the next few days you will be nicotine-free! If you did the Gradual Withdrawal Plan, the level of nicotine in your bloodstream is low and the withdrawal symptoms I'm about to describe should be minimal. This is your reward for your good work in Phase 1! If you did the Cold Turkey Plan, you will be out of withdrawal within the next 24 to 72 hours, so relax!

Let's investigate Nicotine Withdrawal:

CRAVING FOR TOBACCO

You crave tobacco because it contains nicotine, a highly addictive drug that has you chemically hooked. You need it like a heroin addict needs a "fix." If you smoke a pack a day, you need a "fix" every 20 minutes or so. Breathing is the only other thing that you do with such regularity.

When the level of nicotine in your bloodstream begins to drop, the body sends the following message to your brain:

"I need nicotine," which translates to "I need a cigarette."

To help rid your body of nicotine:

- Drink plenty of water and fluids — 6 to 8 glasses or more;
- Sweat out the toxins — Exercise, sauna, jacuzzi, hot bath — helps open the pores and rid your body of the drug;
- Eat organic foods and avoid processed foods high in sugar, preservatives and salt.

DIZZINESS, SPACINESS AND INABILITY TO CONCENTRATE

If you can't find your keys or carry on a conversation, it's because your body chemistry is re-adjusting not only to a drop in nicotine level, but also to an increase in your oxygen supply.

When you smoke, you inhale a gas called carbon monoxide (CO) — the same gas that comes out of your car's tailpipe – which robs your body of oxygen and leaves your brain oxygen-starved. When you quit smoking, your brain receives more oxygen than you're used to, causing lightheadedness.

To best handle these symptoms:

- *Lie down and relax* if you feel dizzy or light-headed;
- *Keep organized* to help you concentrate — ease up on your workload if possible.

IRRITABILITY, ANGER, AND EMOTIONAL REACTIVITY

Feeling emotionally reactive, irritable or testy during withdrawal is normal and understandable.

Quitting smoking is not only a chemical adjustment, but a major psychological adjustment as well.

Although your e-Cigarette and new habit breaking behaviors help, you must learn to cope directly with feelings suppressed by smoking.

To help you remain your usual *nice* self while you adjust emotionally, take a second before speaking to think of **what to say and how to say it.**

Four great communication skills to deal with emotional reactivity (irritability, anger, etc.)

1. Set your intention to have a "solution oriented" conversation (vs. "problem creating");

2. Commit to staying "solution oriented" throughout the entire conversation;

3. Take full responsibility for losing emotional control;

4. Inspire interconnection (Panel 7 — *Light*) by being humble and apologizing immediately.

Stay away from "problem creating" intentions such as:

*   BLAMING – A way of projecting the problem onto another and avoiding responsibility;

*   CRITICIZING – Don't criticize unless you don't mind being criticized;

*   JUDGING – A protective position close to projection which blocks people from approaching you;

*   SARCASM – A passive/aggressive way to hurt others, which might leave you feeling better in the moment, but risks resentment and transparently masks your fear;

*   ARGUMENTS OVER PAST ISSUES – Unless the intention is for resolution (Panel 7 – To Light), not revolution (Panel 6 — Explosions), don't bring up the past.

- USING "YOU" MESSAGES – WATCH YOUR USE OF LANGUAGE. Instead of "you" use "we." For example: Instead of "You did this all wrong," say, "What can we do to make it right?" "We" creates cooperation (Panel 7 — Light) and prevents arguments and negative reactions — "Explosions" (Panel 6).

Note: The only appropriate use of the You Message is when sharing your feelings. Try the "When you...I feel..." format to express yourself.

Example: "When you don't listen, I feel hurt and disconnected from you."

Remember to self reflect and think before you speak, and self correct with an apology if you misspeak. This will maintain high integrity between yourself and others.

Giving up a psychological crutch such as smoking and experiencing withdrawal symptoms can make you anxious. Don't forget that smoking is embedded in every aspect of your life. Quitting can make you feel as if your world is caving in.

It's not.

To help calm your anxiety:

- Take frequent deep breaths; exhale slowly and completely;
- Eat right and take your vitamins to balance your system;
- Try yoga or deep stretching to calm down;
- Listen to calming music;
- Meditate 20 minutes a day at night before going to bed. Clear your mind of all thoughts, relax, give your thinking a rest. The body will follow;
- Maintain a quiet environment as much as possible.

SLEEPINESS OR LACK OF ENERGY

You may feel sleepy and lack energy. As a smoker, you were constantly pumping yourself up, and over stimulating yourself, or slowing yourself down — nicotine has this paradoxical effect.

If you have a hard time falling asleep, the amino acid ***L-tryptophan*** can help. It is good for depression and anxiety as well, and it's available over-the-counter at any drug store. It is also found in turkey, which is why you can often feel sleepy after a big Thanksgiving dinner.

ENERGY CURVE

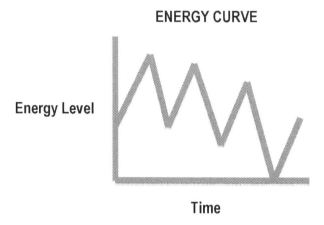

Energy Level

Time

Your first cigarette of the day has powerful effects — nicotine stimulates the central nervous system and the adrenal glands — boosting your energy. Without cigarettes (and coffee), your system tends to feel sluggish.

Twenty minutes after the first "hit," nicotine has a depressant effect, causing you to need a "pick-me-up." This vicious cycle — the rise and fall of your energy, leaves you feeling tired and stressed by the end of the day (see graph above).

When you choose to quit nicotine, you opt out of using the drug to self medicate to boost your energy. To remain balanced, you need to replace your energy source with good nutrition – consider it your healthy "drug."

Refer to your healthy food choices, and re-read FOODS TO AVOID. Here are more suggestions to keep your energy balanced:

The Habit Breakers Quickie Breakfast Idea:

In a blender, mix one cup of:

- non-fat, low-fat, soy, or almond milk
- half a banana, low fat yogurt or protein powder
- fresh or frozen berries (for extra antioxidants,) or any fruit

During The Day Pick-Me-Up:

- Eat instant "fuel foods," such as fresh fruit or whole-grain snacks;

- Protein (an egg, protein bar, nuts, etc.) will help sustain you;

- Eat frequently (small meals every three hours). Don't forget to take your vitamins and minerals.

Reminder: Avoid the following biochemical triggers for nicotine. They set you up for an *energy plunge:*

- Coffee or tea — anything caffeinated;

- Any stimulant drug except by prescription;

- Alcohol;

- Sugar;

- White flour products — refined carbs quickly turn to sugar.

RESTLESSNESS

Cigarettes play a major role in keeping boredom away. If you feel restless before going to sleep: drink a warm glass of milk or an herbal tea such as valerian or chamomile, take one dosage of the amino acid L-tryptophan, or relax into a hot bath.

HEADACHES

Nicotine constricts blood vessels in your brain. As you stop smoking, these vessels will readjust themselves, causing headaches. These headaches will pass shortly. Seek quiet and a darkened room, or lie down for a moment. Only take aspirin or other pain relievers if you absolutely need to.

COUGHING

Smokers often complain that their cough gets worse after quitting. This is normal. Bronchial cilia — hair-like structures along the bronchial passageway which clean your lungs — are paralyzed by smoking. As these cilia heal, the cough disappears. Again, an herbal tea or hot water with lemon and honey helps soothe your throat to arrest the cough reflex, along with a steady flow of menthol or elderberry (sugar-free if possible) cough drops as needed.

MOUTH SORES AND SKIN ODORS

As toxins caused from smoking are naturally released by the body, you may notice mouth, throat or tongue sores and bad breath. This is very common. By stopping the flow of nicotine and other toxic chemicals with your cessation of smoking, you allow your body to cleanse itself, which can result in such sores and odor. Your body has an amazing ability to heal — allow and aid it in this important task. Exercise, take your hot baths and saunas – anything to help you sweat out these toxins.

HUNGER AND WEIGHT GAIN

Quitting smoking doesn't necessarily mean gaining weight. Withdrawing from nicotine may increase your appetite and temporarily decrease your metabolism, slowing down your ability to burn fat. More than a few excess pounds of weight gain is an indication that you've substituted food for cigarettes. Use your suggested cigarette substitutes, increase your exercise, follow your nutritional suggestions, and re-read the section on Weight Control.

CONSTIPATION

Without the stimulant effects of nicotine, your bowels may slow down. Also remember you are releasing toxins through your bowels as well. You may notice a particularly sulfuric smell, indicating this. To help relieve constipation:

- Eat a high-fiber diet — fruits (especially prunes, apricots, kiwi), whole grains (such as high-fiber bread and cereals), nuts and seeds (especially flax) and vegetables (carrots, artichokes, beans);

- Drink plenty of fluids and fresh fruit juice, especially prune, pineapple, papaya and mango — all excellent for your digestive tract;

- Eat Greek yogurt (highest in protein) with berries or the above fruits with organic low-sugar granola or wheat germ;

- Juice vegetables such as beets, carrots, wheat grass, spinach, celery with watermelon, apples, berries etc.

DREAMING THAT YOU'VE SMOKED

Wish Fulfillment through dreams (a theory credited to Dr. Sigmund Freud) is your psyche's way of dealing with your loss. It may persist for weeks. Enjoy — it's the safest cigarette you can smoke!

LESS COMMON SYMPTOMS OF WITHDRAWAL

- GAS OR FLATULENCE: May last several weeks. Avoid foods such as beans, cabbage or cauliflower.

- DIARRHEA: Can last a few days. The body is adjusting to new digestive changes. Water (specially that with electrolytes) and high fiber foods such as oatmeal should help.

- ACID INDIGESTION/HEARTBURN: May increase but will go away. Can last for weeks. Try an over-the-counter antacid and eat well.

- NAUSEA: Usually lasts less than a week. Carbonated mineral water helps. Remember, nausea is the body's natural defense to keep you from eating while there is an infection, or, in your case, toxins, present in the stomach and digestive tract. This is normal and will pass.

Note: If any of the above symptoms cause you undue discomfort, please consult your doctor or medical practitioner.

The graph below is a general description of nicotine withdrawal over time.

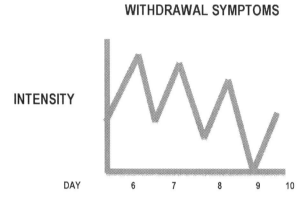

Withdrawal symptoms typically subside within 24 to 72 hours. Everyone responds differently. If you've spent 5 days weaning off nicotine, it should decrease your timeline significantly. If you are on the Cold Turkey Plan, you should feel relief within a few days.

At Day 6 your craving for nicotine is at its highest point and your control is at its lowest. By Day 8 or 9 (or probably sooner if you've weaned yourself off the drug), you will begin to experience symptom relief.

You may find that your withdrawal symptoms get worse before they get better. Worry not. This is an indication that your body is almost nicotine free! It's a very positive sign.

BREAKING THE POSITIVE ASSOCIATIONS WITH SMOKING: REWIRING THE CONNECTIONS

Remember your first cigarette? Remember the coughing, the dizziness, and the nausea? Your gut told you that there was...something wrong. You forced yourself to get past the negative feelings and trained yourself to enjoy smoking. You will now need to do this again... for a positive result.

According to brain researchers, neurons (pleasure pathways in the brain) that fire together, wire together.

By associating breathing, relaxing, and rewarding yourself with smoking, you created positive associations with your habit, reinforced your addiction to nicotine, and wired, or "encoded" the habit (see Panel 3 — Encoding).

Today you will begin to rewire your positive associations, replace them with negative ones, and break up this deadly love affair (Panel 4 — Letting Go).

RECORD 5 POSITIVE AND 5 NEGATIVE ASSOCIATIONS WITH SMOKING.

SMOKING'S "TURN ONS:"

1. _____

2. _____

3. _____

4. _____

5. _____

SMOKING'S "TURN OFFS:"

1. _____

2. _____

3. _____

4. _____

5. _____

COUNTER-CONDITIONING EXERCISE: TURNING OFF TO SMOKING

You will now begin rewiring your positive associations with smoking and replacing them with negative sensations such as coughing, congestion, stale smell and bitter taste. This exercise helps you kick the habit on a "gut-level," and lose the desire to smoke (remember, you can't be talked out of a habit).

It is called "counter-conditioning."

OPEN YOUR PACK OF CIGARETTES AND LIGHT UP

Inhale. Take a few seconds to think about what you enjoy about this puff on your cigarette. Is it the taste, smell, warmth, smoke, sucking motion, feeling in your chest, the high from the drug?

WRITE DOWN THE 3 MOST ENJOYABLE ASPECTS OF THIS PUFF

1. _____

2. _____

3. _____

For the next 10 puffs, image that your body is allergic to the smoke. As you smoke, imagine the sooty, tarry smoke cutting off your oxygen supply, coating your lung tissue with poisons. Imagine that you're suffocating and can barely breathe.

Note the negative feelings associated with these realistic, damaging facts. Notice how you're killing yourself.

Now proceed as you smoke to rewire the messages. In the following exercise you are activating Panel 4 — Letting Go — and consciously breaking the old bonds that once enslaved you to your habit and addiction.

COUNTER-CONDITIONING EXERCISE:

1. Inhale and cough up the smoke. Your mouth is beginning to taste bitter.

2. Inhale and cough it up again. The bitter flavor is getting stronger and your throat feels dry and scratchy.

3. Inhale and cough. Your throat feels tight and dry, and your chest feels congested.

4. Inhale and cough. Picture the heavy tarry smoke sitting in your chest, pressing down on you like a ton of bricks.

5. Inhale and cough. Your chest feels tight, and you're having trouble breathing.

6. Inhale and cough. Your chest feels congested and you can hardly breathe.

7. Inhale and cough. You can feel a tight lump at the back of your throat and your lungs feel raw and irritated.

8. Inhale and cough. Your throat feels raw; your chest feels heavy; and you can barely squeeze the smoke down into your chest.

9. Inhale and cough it up – hard.

10. Inhale and cough it up again – harder!

If you still have a strong urge to smoke, repeat this exercise. If you feel sick, stop. When you're ready, throw your cigarette butts and your unused cigarettes into the jar of water. Save one cigarette for the next exercise.

Note: Discarding your unused cigarettes rewires your brain to perceive your once highly valued cigarettes as having zero value.

TRANSFERRING THE PLEASURE OF SMOKING TO e-SMOKING

Keep the pleasure, lose the pain...

WARNING: If you are pregnant, or suspect that you are, if you have a history of health problems such as heart disease, high blood pressure, stroke, emphysema, hyper or hypoglycemia, or any other serious health problem, follow the instructions below, but do not inhale the smoke into your lungs (except for the first inhalation). Instead, inhale to the back of your throat only for the rest of the exercise. If you experience dizziness, lightheadedness or heart palpitations, stop immediately. For questions or concerns about the counter-conditioning exercises, consult your doctor or medical practitioner.

Your e-Cigarette allows you to keep the pleasure of smoking and lose the pain (the harmful side effects). It's your Fantasy Cigarette come true!

Your e-Cigarette is an important transitional object. It creates a bridge from addiction to freedom and helps you stay more calm and balanced while you adjust to your new non-smoking lifestyle. As you switch back and forth between the cigarette and the e-Cigarette, you retrain yourself to transfer the pleasure from Smoking to e-Smoking.

READ FIRST BEFORE DOING THIS EXERCISE

- Light up a cigarette and hold it in the opposite hand you use to smoke;
- Hold your e-Cigarette in the hand you use to smoke;
- Inhale one puff of the cigarette. Look for it's "turn offs" and mentally rate the pleasure on a 1-10 scale;
- Inhale one puff of the e-Cigarette. Look for its "turn ons" and mentally rate the pleasure on a 1-10 scale;
- For the next 10 puffs, switch back and forth between the two. Keep mentally rating the pleasure (1-10 scale) and deliberately focus your attention on the harsh, bitter, negative sensations of the cigarette verses the light, refreshing positive sensations of your e-Cigarette;

- If, after 10 puffs, the cigarette still tastes better than the e-Cigarette, redo this exercise for 10 puffs. This time, cough up each inhale on the cigarette and work actively to counter-condition yourself to "turn off" to smoking cigarettes. Remember, you have to be an active participant in your success.

NOTE: When you're ready, throw your cigarette butts and your unused cigarettes into the jar of water, wash up, brush your teeth, rinse your mouth, and continue reading when you're done.

EASING NICOTINE CRAVINGS

To help you when nicotine cravings are more intense, here are 3 easy coping skills:

1. FOCAL POINT BREATHING TECHNIQUE

Focal Point Breathing is an adaptation of the Lamaze Technique, a pain management technique used to ease the pain of childbirth. It works equally effectively to take the focus off nicotine cravings.

Here's how to do it:

Find a comfortable spot to sit or lie down;

- Choose a focal point — a specific spot comfortably above eye level. Focus your attention there;

- When the craving hits, breathe in deeply through your nose (or mouth if that's more comfortable), project your craving onto your focal point. Say to yourself **"Hello, craving. Welcome *in.*"**

- As you exhale slowly through your mouth, imagine that you are *pushing the craving away,* into space. Say to yourself, **"Goodbye craving. Thanks for passing *through.*"**

There is a great saying that applies here: *"Resistance is Persistence."* By your ability to **stop resisting** the craving, you can flow with it and allow it to pass *through* you. Practice your ability to dispose of your urges through *Focal Point Breathing*.

75

2. "GROUNDING" THE CRAVING" BREATHING TECHNIQUE

Grounding The Craving is like discharging static electricity build-up in your body.

Here's how it works:

- Sit comfortably in a chair, uncross your arms and legs, and plant your feet on the ground;

- When you feel a craving, inhale through your nose, and imagine sending the breath to the top of your head;

- As you exhale, imagine gathering up your craving with your breath, sending it down your body into the soles of your feet and grounding your craving into the floor.

Keep cleaning and discharging your cravings in this way so they don't cause stress build-up. Smoking used to cue you to breathe deeply. Now that you're not, remind yourself to frequently breathe deep on your own. Fortunately, you're only giving up smoking — not breathing!

SENSE MEMORY TECHNIQUE

Sense Memory is a way to recall memories of sensations. Use it to recreate the memory of your most recent experience with smoking's "turn offs."

Here's how:

- Whenever you have a craving to smoke, close your eyes, and recall the 3 most potent negative sensations about your smoking experience (such as the harsh bitter taste, coughing, irritation, etc.);

- Lock in the Sense Memory by squeezing your fist every time you "get" the feeling – as if trapping it into the palm of your hand;

- Let these sensations hit you on a "gut level." You'll know that you got it when you can feel it.

IMPORTANT REMINDER:

ONE THOUGHT RE-ADDICTS: NEVER FLIRT WITH YOUR DESIRE TO SMOKE!

It's a mental trick that will sabotage you back to smoking. Instead, rewire your desire and <u>kill it</u> with your Sense Memory Technique. Practice it as many times as you have a craving.

<u>ONE PUFF RE-ADDICTS</u>: <u>NEVER SMOKE BETWEEN SESSIONS</u>!

<u>One puff</u> on a cigarette (other than when instructed to do so in the exercises) will re-addict you to smoking!

Note: Use your Quitter's Survival Guide (refer to it often) for quick helpful reminders about quitting.

You're well on your way to breaking free from your habit and addiction. You are on Panel 4 – "Letting Go." The old, positive associations you built up with smoking are breaking. Why? Because you caused them to break through your positive intentions and hard work. There is a lot of freedom in Letting Go.

TOMORROW'S SUPPLIES:

ONE PACK OF YOUR LEAST FAVORITE BRAND OF CIGARETTES (DON'T BUY THEM UNTIL RIGHT BEFORE YOUR SESSION AND DON'T OPEN THE PACK UNTIL YOU ARE INSTRUCTED TO DO SO), GLASS JAR WITH WATER, LIGHER OR MATCHES, AND A WATCH OR CLOCK WITH A 'SECONDS' HAND.

PLEASE SIGN YOUR DAY 6 CONTRACT AND RETURN TOMORROW AT YOUR SCHEDULED TIME.

PHASE 2: COLD TURKEY

HABIT BREAKERS COLD TURKEY

STOP SMOKING CONTRACT FOR KICK IT! DAY 6

I _____, commit to quitting smoking cigarettes permanently. I agree to temporarily transfer my nicotine addiction from cigarettes to my e-Cigarette as I wean off smoking and learn to break the habit and addiction over the course of the 10 Day Plan.

I agree to follow the nicotine dosage schedule below:

- Kick It! Day 6: Switch to smoking your e-Cigarette – Zero mg nicotine filter, flavor only.

I understand and agree that I will not "cheat" and smoke cigarettes during the course of Day 6 (or at any other time for that matter), or use nicotine replacement therapy (NRT — gums, patches, or any other form of nicotine, etc.) to supplement my cravings.

I understand that the above dosages are most likely less than I am accustomed to ingesting, and that my withdrawal symptoms began as soon as I made the dosage switch from smoking cigarettes to e-Smoking.

I understand that the experience of withdrawal varies from person to person, that they are temporary, and that I can refer to the section on HOW TO HANDLE NICOTINE WITHDRAWAL—Kick It! Day 6, as needed.

I understand that by choosing the Gradual Withdrawal Plan, I have prepared my body to have an easier withdrawal experience for Cold Turkey Phase 2.

I agree to rid my environment of tobacco, cigarettes, matches, lighters, ashtrays, and other smoking paraphernalia.

I am quitting smoking for myself, and of my own free will and I'm choosing to do so for the following reasons:

MY 5 MOST IMPORTANT BENEFITS OF QUITTING:

1. _____

2. _____

3. _____

4. _____

5. _____

Signed _____

Dated _____

PHASE 2: COLD TURKEY

KICK IT! DAY 7: TRANSFORMING YOUR RELATIONSHIP WITH SMOKING

PLEASE CONTINUE TO SMOKING YOUR e-CIGARETTE — ZERO MG NICOTINE, FLAVOR ONLY FILTER

Reminder:

- Rid your environment of cigarettes, all forms of tobacco and all smoking paraphernalia — matches, lighters, ashtrays, etc.

HOMEWORK: PLEASE READ *NOW*

Important: Don't open your pack of cigarettes until you are instructed to smoke. It's vital to the success of the Plan that you wait for instructions.

Congratulations, ex-smoker! You've made it through the first 24 hours without nicotine. By now you're probably anxious to smoke those cigarettes you just picked up from the store. You are still going through withdrawal, and most likely missing nicotine. In just a few minutes, you'll have a chance to smoke your cigarettes — "turn off" style, of course.

Yesterday, we talked about the positive associations you built up with smoking and how these positive associations were initially created.

The best puff on a cigarette is usually the first puff. It's because the relaxing effects of oxygen kick in before the nicotine and carbon monoxide (CO) poisons. The first puff fools you into thinking that smoking is relaxing.

It's only later, after you extinguish your cigarette, that you begin to feel uncomfortable. When the nicotine content in your blood level drops, another false association is formed: Your mind concludes that not smoking is irritating and never makes the connection that smoking causes the discomfort of withdrawal symptoms in the first place. This is because there is no direct connection between the irritation and the cigarette — the cigarette is already out by the time the irritation sets in!

That's how you end up with these two false associations (mental equations):

Smoking = Relaxation and Not Smoking = Irritation

Today you're going to allow your body to *direct connect* with the smoking-induced irritation by *bypassing* your feelings of relaxation.

Because you haven't smoked for 24 hours, you are extremely sensitive to nicotine and will experience <u>full on</u> how this drug is killing you! Partaking in today's counter-conditioning exercise will activate Panel 6 — "Explosions." This time, for good cause: To launch a war against your habit and addiction. Your weapon — your cigarette!

PHYSIOLOGICAL EFFECTS OF SMOKING: NICOTINE POISONING

Here's how nicotine poisoning affects you:

- Your heart rate increases. Smoking stimulates certain glands to release adrenalin and powerful hormones, causing the walls of the heart to contract, increasing your heart rate and need for oxygen;

- Your blood vessels constrict, increasing your blood pressure, and restricts blood flow to your outer extremities, leaving you with cold, tingly sensations in your fingers and toes;

- Your oxygen supply decreases. Carbon monoxide (CO), which makes up about 4% of cigarette smoke, robs your bloodstream of oxygen. It attracts red blood cells (which distribute oxygen throughout the body) stronger than oxygen, blocking oxygen absorption. This impairs your vision, attention to sound, athletic performance, good judgment and ability to think clearly. It can also cause you to feel spacey and dizzy.

- Stomach acid level increases. Nicotine raises your blood sugar level, which fools your body into sensing that you've just eaten, and interferes with your stomach's ability to buffer acid, causing you to feel nauseous.

Imagine what 20 cigarettes a day does to your stomach lining! That's why so many smokers develop ulcers.

TAKE YOUR RESTING PULSE

Before you begin your counter-conditioning exercise:

- Find a good strong pulse spot on your wrist (below the thumb is a good spot);

- Take your pulse for 10 seconds and multiply this number by 6 to calculate your heartbeats/minute (example: a count of 12 beats/10 seconds x 6 =72);

- Record your resting pulse rate.

_____ x 6 = _____
pulse/10 seconds   resting heart rate

The rapid inhalation of smoke (as instructed in this exercise) is a very effective tool to help you induce low level of nicotine poisoning and break your positive associations with nicotine. But it may be bad for you.

WARNING: <u>ALTERNATIVE EXERCISE</u>: If you are pregnant, or suspect that you are, if you have a history of health problems such as heart disease, high blood pressure, stroke, emphysema, hyper or hypoglycemia, or any other serious health problem, follow the instructions below, but do not inhale the smoke into your lungs (except for the first inhalation). Instead, inhale to the back of your throat <u>only</u> for the rest of the exercise. If you experience dizziness, lightheadedness or heart palpitations, stop immediately. For questions or concerns about the counter-conditioning exercises, consult your doctor or medical practitioner.

RAPID SMOKING COUNTER-CONDITIONING EXERCISE

For the duration of one cigarette, you will inhale every 7 seconds as you look for signs of increased heart rate, tingling in the extremities, light-headedness, dizziness, nausea and acid stomach.

Stop smoking as soon as you feel some of these physiological effects.

If you feel faint or ill, stop the exercise immediately and continue with the alternate counter-conditioning exercise.

Take out a cigarette, break off the filter, light up, and start inhaling every 7 seconds as you do and say the following:

1. Inhale and cough up the smoke. "I'm poisoning my body with nicotine."

2. Inhale and cough it up again. "Nicotine has hit my brain, and I can feel the effects of the drug."

3. Inhale and cough. "My head feels dizzy from the lack of oxygen and effects of carbon monoxide."

4. Inhale and cough. "I feel lightheaded and drugged."

5. Inhale and cough. "My heart is starting to beat harder and faster."

6. Inhale and cough. "My fingers and toes feel cold and tingly."

7. Inhale and cough. "I feel light-headed and dizzy."

8. Inhale and cough. "My stomach feels queasy."

9. Inhale and cough it up – hard. "I'm starting to feel a bit nauseous."

10. Inhale and cough it up again – harder! "Cigarettes are beginning to lose some of their power over me."

If you still have a strong urge to smoke, repeat this exercise. Stop if you feel sick. ***When you're ready, throw your cigarette butts and your unused cigarettes into the jar of water.***

Take your pulse rate again and record it here: _____

Take your resting pulse rate/minute and subtract it from your rapid pulse rate after smoking.

_____ - _____ = _____

pulse/per minute   after smoking pulse/per minute   difference

To get the percentage increase, take the difference between the two rates and divide it by your resting pulse.

_____ -:- _____ = _____

       difference   resting pulse/per minute   % increase

Most smokers show a 20% to 30% increase in pulse rate after smoking. Heavy smokers initially show a decrease in heart rate. These nicotine-induced changes put a big strain on the heart. In fact, every year cigarette smoking is a factor in 120,000 U.S. deaths from coronary heart disease. Stop smoking and you've reduced your chances of being a statistic.

If you still have a strong urge to smoke, repeat this exercise. If you feel sick, stop. When you're ready, throw your cigarette butts and your unused cigarettes into the jar of water.

Note: Discarding your unused cigarettes rewires your brain to perceive your once highly valued cigarettes as having zero value.

It hurts to see all that money gone down the toilet, doesn't it? Ask yourself honestly if you'd rather the smoke go down into your lungs instead. Wash up, brush your teeth, drink some water, and RETURN back here when you're done.

MORE ON SMOKING, PREGNANCY, AND ITS EFFECTS ON YOUR FETUS AND CHILD

If nicotine poisoning made you sick, imagine its effects on your fetus and/or child!

- More and more studies show that smoking during pregnancy has a significantly adverse effect upon the well-being of the fetus, the health of the newborn baby, and the future development of the infant into childhood;
- Women who smoke during pregnancy have significantly more stillbirths;
- More babies of smoking mothers die during the first month of infancy than those who do not smoke;
- 20% of unsuccessful pregnancies might have been successful if the mother had not been a regular smoker;
- Babies of smoking mothers weigh about 6 ounces less that those of non-smoking mothers. The more a woman smokes

during pregnancy, the less her infant will weigh. The earlier a woman gives up smoking during pregnancy, the less her risk of delivering a low birth-weight baby;

- When a pregnant woman smokes, the amount of carbon monoxide (CO) in the blood increases, depleting her fetus of oxygen;

- Pediatricians have found that children of parents who smoke have more upper respiratory and ear infections than those of non-smoking parents;

- Long-term follow-up studies show that children of mothers who smoked heavily during pregnancy are shorter in stature, have retarded reading ability, and lower ratings on social adjustment than the children of non-smoking mothers;

- Parents who smoke role model to their children that the behavior of smoking is acceptable. Children mimic a parent's behavior and ignore any preaching the parents don't practice. Children of smokers are twice as likely to start smoking as are children of non-smokers.

Without a doubt, quitting smoking is the most significant gift you can give your child.

IMPORTANT REMINDERS:

ONE THOUGHT RE-ADDICTS: NEVER FLIRT WITH YOUR DESIRE TO SMOKE! It's a mental trick that will sabotage you back to smoking. Instead, rewire your desire and <u>kill it</u> with your Sense Memory Technique. Practice it as many times as you have a craving.

ONE PUFF RE-ADDICTS: NEVER SMOKE BETWEEN SESSIONS! <u>One puff</u> on a cigarette (other than when instructed to do so in the exercises) will re-addict you by turning you back "on" to smoking!

Note: Use your Quitter's Survival Guide (refer to it often) for quick helpful reminders about quitting.

TOMORROW'S SUPPLIES:

ONE PACK OF YOUR LEAST FAVORITE BRAND OF CIGARETTES (DON'T BUY THEM UNTIL RIGHT BEFORE YOUR SESSION AND DON'T OPEN THE PACK UNTIL YOU ARE INSTRUCTED TO DO SO), GLASS JAR WITH WATER, LIGHER OR MATCHES, AND A WATCH OR CLOCK WITH A 'SECONDS' HAND.

PLEASE SIGN YOUR DAY 7 CONTRACT AND RETURN TOMORROW AT YOUR SCHEDULED TIME.

PHASE 2: COLD TURKEY

HABIT BREAKERS COLD TURKEY

STOP SMOKING CONTRACT FOR KICK IT! DAY 7

I _____, commit to quitting smoking cigarettes permanently. I agree to temporarily transfer my nicotine addiction from cigarettes to my e-Cigarette as I wean off smoking and learn to break the habit and addiction over the course of the 10 Day Plan.

I agree to follow the nicotine dosage schedule below:

- Kick It! Day 7: Continue smoking your e-Cigarette – Zero mg nicotine filter, flavor only.

I understand and agree that I will not "cheat" and smoke cigarettes during the course of Day 7 (or at any other time for that matter), or use nicotine replacement therapy (NRT — gums, patches, or any other form of nicotine, etc.) to supplement my cravings.

I understand that the above dosages are most likely less than I am accustomed to ingesting, and that my withdrawal symptoms began as soon as I made the dosage switch from smoking cigarettes to e-Smoking.

I understand that the experience of withdrawal varies from person to person, that they are temporary, and that I can refer to the section on HOW TO HANDLE NICOTINE WITHDRAWAL—Kick It! Day 6, as needed.

I understand that by choosing the Gradual Withdrawal Plan, I have prepared my body to have an easier withdrawal experience for Cold Turkey Phase 2.

I agree to rid my environment of tobacco, cigarettes, matches, lighters, ashtrays, and other smoking paraphernalia.

I am quitting smoking for myself, and of my own free will and I'm choosing to do so for the following reasons:

MY 5 MOST IMPORTANT BENEFITS OF QUITTING:

1. _____

2. _____

3. _____

4. _____

5. _____

Signed _____

Dated _____

PHASE 2: COLD TURKEY

KICK IT! DAY 8: WHY ONE PUFF RE-ADDICTS

PLEASE CONTINUE TO SMOKING YOUR e-CIGARETTE — ZERO MG NICOTINE, FLAVOR ONLY FILTER

Reminder:

- Rid your environment of cigarettes, all forms of tobacco and all smoking paraphernalia — matches, lighters, ashtrays, etc.

HOMEWORK: PLEASE READ *NOW*

Important: <u>Don't open your pack of cigarettes until you are instructed to smoke</u>. It's vital to the success of the program that you wait for instructions.

Congratulations, ex-smoker! You made it through your second 24 hours without nicotine!

You've certainly heard it enough times and seen enough examples from either your own past attempts at quitting or someone else's experience with relapse: One puff re-addicts.

You may be wondering why, if one puff re-addicts, I have you smoke during your Plan, and why those cigarettes don't re-addict you to smoking.

The answer: One puff re-addicts you psychologically, not chemically. To re-addict yourself chemically, you would need to smoke more than what you smoke during your sessions, and you would have to smoke "turn on" style to re-addict yourself back into the habit and addiction. Let me illustrate with an example from animal research.

THE RAT RACE & THE HUMAN RACE

One of the most influential figures in modern psychology is Behavioral Psychologist B.F. Skinner. One of his early contributions to behavioral psychology was the "Skinner Box" – designed to study an animal's learning ability.

When a rat is placed in it and pushes a lever, a mechanism delivers a pellet of food to the animal. The Skinner Box makes it possible to study different reward systems and their influence on animal behavior.

CONTINUOUS REINFORCEMENT

A rat has been taught to bar-press a food lever to obtain food. Each time the rat presses the lever, a food pellet falls out. That's called continuous reinforcement — 100% of the rat's lever-pressing leads to the food reward.

Let's say that this rat has been busily pressing away and eating for months, and suddenly the experimenter shuts off the food reward "cold turkey." Assuming that the rat is fed outside the cage so that it doesn't starve to death, how long do you think it would take for this rat to quit the bar-pressing habit?

Not long.

Within 2 to 3 days the rat gives up the bar-pressing behavior. The "cold turkey" method kills the habit quickly.

INTERMITTENT, OR PARTIAL REINFORCEMENT

Let's look at another situation. What would happen if just before the rat gives up bar-pressing, a food pellet falls out?

He would not only regain hope in the system, he would press the lever harder and more frequently than ever! This schedule of reinforcement is called Intermittent, or Partial Reinforcement. It's the strongest reinforcement schedule for developing habits.

Let's plug you into this scenario. As a smoker, just about every time you wanted a cigarette, you got one. Your urges to smoke were reinforced 100% of the time. When you started Phase 2 of your Plan you were asked to stop smoking nicotine Cold Turkey. You were only permitted to smoke "turn off" style, which was neither rewarding nor psychologically reinforcing. That's why it didn't re-addict you.

By remaining on the Cold Turkey schedule, your urge to smoke will fade relatively quickly – just like the rat's bar pressing habit was broken when the behavior was no longer reinforced. <u>Any habit that isn't rewarded or reinforced fades over time</u>.

What if you gave in to "just one puff" on a cigarette? I think you already know. It would "re-ignite" your smoking habit and wipe out all the negative associations you've built up, reinforce all the urges that made you give in and take that puff. You'd develop amnesia as to why you stopped smoking in the first place!

<u>You can't be a part-time smoker</u>. If you think you can, you're dreaming, or worse – lying to yourself. It's an <u>all or nothing</u> commitment.

Here's why: If you say "No" a thousand times to smoking, and then finally give in with one "Yes," you reinforce those <u>thousand</u> urges with that <u>one</u> puff on a cigarette. Not only do you re-addict yourself, but you strengthen your habit. Look again at Panel 3 — "Encoding." Smoking "just one puff" reinforces the bonds that bind you to the habit and worse, strengthens them!

That "one puff" will bring you back to smoking the same amount you smoked before you quit, and will quickly escalates into one pack, two packs, five packs... or whatever satisfied your usual daily need.

One last point before you open your pack of cigarettes: The obvious difference between you and the rat in the above example is that the rat has no choice. As humans, we always have a choice – to smoke, or not to smoke.

If you want to have an easy time as an ex-smoker, you can do it by choosing to create a "no-hope" consciousness, or "no-hope" attitude. Go back to Panel 1 — Darkness, and bring Darkness to "hope."

That's right. Don't give yourself any "hope" of smoking after today's session. If you experience a craving, nip it in the bud immediately. <u>Do not build up a desire for the cigarette by flirting with it and falling in love again</u>.

When you adopt a "no-hope" or "no-chance-for-a-cigarette" attitude, you are telling your mind that you have predetermined the issue of whether or not you smoke and that's it's <u>not up for discussion</u>. "Hope" is the breeding ground for cravings. Give it up and your cravings will disappear.

Chemically, it takes about 48 to 72 hours for your body to rid itself of nicotine. Psychologically, it takes about 21 days to change a habit. Stick with it. With time it gets easier and easier to stay off cigarettes.

Today is your last day of smoking. By tomorrow 72 hours will have passed and you will be out of withdrawal. Please remember that each individual's reaction time differs. If you are still experiencing withdrawal symptoms, give it a little more time. You'll come out of it very soon.

Ready for a cigarette? I wouldn't be surprised if you're still anxious to smoke. Of course you are. You're still chemically addicted. You still need your "fix."

COUNTER-CONDTIONING EXERCISE:
BREAKING THE POSITIVE IMAGE OF SMOKING

It's time to become aware of how you look when you smoke. Let's re-examine the image you portray as a smoker.

NOTE: Today you will watch yourself smoke in a mirror — find one.

Please open your pack of cigarettes.

To warm up, light your cigarette, inhale, and cough up the smoke. Do this 3 times. From this point on you will be puffing without inhaling on 2 cigarettes at a time. Watch yourself in the mirror as you puff away on your favorite pacifier. Keep puffing until you're done with these 2 cigarettes, then light up 2 more and continue to puff on them until they're finished.

Stop and look at yourself in the mirror. Look familiar? Remember the last time you were at a party full of smokers and you chain-smoked through the drinks? Remember when you stayed up late to finish a project and smoked until your eyes turned bloodshot red?

Notice the taste in your mouth; also the smell of smoke in your hair and clothes – familiar?

Take out an unlit cigarette and <u>without</u> lighting up, go through the motions of inhaling and exhaling as you watch yourself in the mirror.

What does the body language of smoking convey to your children, your lover, your co-workers, to you? Think about this as you continue to watch yourself in the mirror going through the motions of smoking.

Smokers assume awkward positions when holding a cigarette. They either lean away from the smoke or hold their arm away so the smoke doesn't bother them or others. Do you hunch over? Do you curl up?

How does smoking affect your posture? Look in the mirror?

You've now spent two sessions building negative associations with smoking. You have stored many negative sensations in your Sense Memory Bank from your past smoking sessions.

Today, you've had an opportunity to look closer at the visual 'turn offs' of this habit. You can no longer hide behind the belief that smoking is attractive, sexy, relaxing, refreshing, or a harmless habit that only affects "the other guy."

There is no more purpose to smoking beyond this session. It's time to say goodbye to smoking once and for all.

FINAL COUNTER CONDITIONING EXERCISE:

Take out your <u>last</u> cigarette, and light up. You will be inhaling and coughing up your <u>last</u> 10 puffs of a cigarette as you say the following:

1. Inhale and cough. "Smoking makes my lips burn."

2. Inhale and cough. "Smoking irritates my eyes."

3. Inhale and cough. "Smoking irritates my throat and makes it feel scratchy and uncomfortable."

4. Inhale and cough. "Smoking makes my chest feel heavy and congested."

5. Inhale and cough. "Smoking irritates my nose and causes my nose to feel dry and itchy."

6. Inhale and cough. "Smoking makes my stomach queasy."

7. Inhale and cough. "Smoking makes my head feel tight."

8. Inhale and cough. "Smoking puts my nerves on edge."

9. Inhale and cough. "Smoking makes me cough."

10. Inhale and cough it up for the last time. "Smoking makes me feel sick and dirty and I won't allow this habit to control me any longer. Goodbye! I'm glad to be done with this habit once and for all!"

Congratulations! You just smoked your last cigarette! You'll never have to abuse your body again!

You've also just completed the middle row of the Mind Map, (Panels 4-6), going "Through" — Withdrawal and Stopping Smoking. Tomorrow you will enter the last phase of your process, the Mind Map's bottom row, (Panels 7-9): "To" — Healing and Freedom.

When you're ready, throw your cigarette butts and your unused cigarettes into the jar of water.

Wash up, brush your teeth, drink some water, and RETURN back here when you're done.

Read this first and get a sense of the visual imagery before beginning your Journey:

VISUALIZATION: JOURNEY THROUGH YOUR MIND MAP

"From" Addiction, "Through" Withdrawal and Stopping Smoking: Panels 1-6

Let's revisit your Mind Map From Addiction Through Withdrawal and Stopping Smoking (Panels 1-6).

Before you begin:

Close your eyes, and take a deep breath in through your nose. Exhale slowly, through your mouth. Now start the exercise.

As you continue to breathe, visualize ocean waves, cleansing, soothing, and washing away the remnants of built-up tar and poisons from your body.

Visualize every breath filling you with energy, vigor and health as you let go of your habit and addiction. Let the waves wash away any fond memories of smoking.

As your body begins to cleanse and relax, you will find yourself breathing more deeply.

Let's begin.

Observe the 9 Panels of the Mind Map in front of you.

See yourself standing in Panel 1 — Darkness, remembering your first unconscious intention to start smoking.

Move to Panel 2 — Manifestation. Run a movie in your head of your past life as a smoker. See how your habit and addiction manifested in every aspect of your life; lighting up first thing in the morning, after a meal, while working, socializing, coping with stress, etc.

Move to Panel 3 — Encoding. Feel the DNA strand twisting and turning around you, entrapping you into the power of the habit and addiction, dictating to you when and how much to smoke.

Move to Panel 4 — Letting Go. Focus your intention on breaking the chains of your habit and addiction once and for all. Feel them release their grasp and fall away.

Move to Panel 5 — Defense Mechanisms. Feel how much and for how long you held in your feelings to protect yourself from losing control and exploding (or imploding).

Move to Panel 6 — Explosions. Feel the defended feelings come to a head and release. Cry, scream, rage if you want to. You are free to self express.

You are at a new Precipice — the Precipice of Healing and Freedom (Panels 7-9). You are more empowered and balanced.

As you take another deep breath, notice how the effects of today's counter-conditioning exercise have almost completely faded.

Tonight, when you go to sleep, visualize the ocean, washing away any remaining positive associations with smoking. Think about how far you've come on your journey, now freeing yourself from your habit and addiction.

When you have an urge to smoke, use your Sense Memory Technique to recall the nauseous effects you experienced in today's session.

PREVENTION: HOW EX-SMOKERS RELAPSE

I want to give you some examples of how quitters re-addict themselves and fall off the wagon. I want you to learn relapse prevention skills so that you can be prepared for any life event.

THE DRINKER

The Drinker tends to forget commitments easily under the influence of alcohol, saying to himself: "Aw, what the heck, one little drink can't really hurt."

When you drink, your strongest resolve disappears. Don't fall into the trap of re-addicting yourself over a glass of booze. If you're going to drink alcohol, drink only in the company of nonsmokers, and not for at least one month after your Habit Breakers Kick It! Day.

Play it safe — avoid alcohol and other non-prescription drugs for as long as you can. Why take chances with your success?

THE CURIOUS TASTER

The Curious Taster fools him/herself into believing they're not really smoking and goes around lighting others' cigarettes, saying, "I don't smoke anymore. I just enjoy the act of lighting up my friend's cigarettes for them."

The Curious Taster is the sort of person who thinks it's cute to show off how much control they have over smoking. Unfortunately, just one puff and the cigarette will re-addict The Curious Taster. Don't be one.

The only safe cigarette is the un-smoked cigarette. The only way to control this addiction is to stay clear of trouble. Don't be a wise-guy at your own expense. Save the tasting for the smokers. You are an ex-smoker, remember?

THE PROGRAM TESTER

The Program Tester reminds me of The Curious Taster, but is much more psychologically sophisticated.

The Program Tester has the Plan all figured out and wants to test to see if he/she is still 'turned off' to smoking — out to prove the Plan wrong — and show that they can "outsmart the system." The Program Tester is very successful at outsmarting...themselves. They return back to smoking again.

THE SPECIAL OCCASION SMOKER

The Special Occasion Smoker feels cheated out of his favorite reward in life – cigarettes. He's the type who wants his cake and eat it too — he wants to smoke only on <u>special occasions</u>, yet wants to remain an ex-smoker.

The Special Occasion Smoker saves those special puffs for special moments: after a romantic meal; to celebrate a special event, etc. It's his special reward, his special personal gift.

The problem with The Special Occasion Smoker is that after taking that one special occasion puff, he often returns to smoking just as much as he did before.

Remember — <u>one puff fully re-addicts you to smoking</u> the same amount you smoked before. You can't be a little bit of a smoker any more than you can be a little bit pregnant. Either you smoke, or you don't.

Forewarned is Forearmed. Savor these special occasions to celebrate your continuing success as a strong and healthy <u>ex-smoker</u>.

REFLECTIONS ON THE ABOVE

These previous counter-conditioning exercises are designed to turn you off to smoking. You don't need to be psychologically sophisticated to know that if you smoke a cigarette, you are looking to enjoy it, not to turn yourself off to it.

If you want to know whether you will always be turned off to smoking, the answer is...NO. Not if you have one puff of it! You will only stay turned off to smoking if you reinforce the negative sensations you experienced in your counter-conditioning sessions. Don't let your addict thinking sabotage you into smoking again.

I would rather you laugh at these characters now than have you experience a relapse with smoking. The more aware you are of these potential traps for failure, the stronger a position you'll be in to say NO to smoking for good.

IMPORTANT REMINDERS:

<u>ONE THOUGHT RE-ADDICTS</u>: NEVER FLIRT WITH YOUR DESIRE TO SMOKE! It's a mental trick that will sabotage you back to smoking. Instead, rewire your desire and <u>kill it</u> with your Sense Memory Technique. Practice it as many times as you have a craving.

<u>ONE PUFF RE-ADDICTS</u>: NEVER SMOKE BETWEEN SESSIONS! <u>One puff</u> on a cigarette (other than when instructed to do so in the exercises) will re-addict you by turning you back "on" to smoking!

Note: Use your Quitter's Survival Guide (refer to it often) for quick helpful reminders about quitting.

PLEASE SIGN YOUR DAY 8 CONTRACT AND RETURN TOMORROW AT YOUR SCHEDULED TIME.

PHASE 2: COLD TURKEY

HABIT BREAKERS COLD TURKEY

STOP SMOKING CONTRACT FOR KICK IT! DAY 8

I _____, commit to quitting smoking cigarettes permanently. I agree to temporarily transfer my nicotine addiction from cigarettes to my e-Cigarette as I wean off smoking and learn to break the habit and addiction over the course of the 10 Day Plan.

I agree to follow the nicotine dosage schedule below:

- Kick It! Day 8: Continue smoking your e-Cigarette – Zero mg nicotine filter, flavor only.

I understand and agree that I will not "cheat" and smoke cigarettes during the course of Day 8 (or at any other time for that matter), or use nicotine replacement therapy (NRT — gums, patches, or any other form of nicotine, etc.) to supplement my cravings.

I understand that the above dosages are most likely less than I am accustomed to ingesting, and that my withdrawal symptoms began as soon as I made the dosage switch from smoking cigarettes to e-Smoking.

I understand that the experience of withdrawal varies from person to person, that they are temporary, and that I can refer to the section on HOW TO HANDLE NICOTINE WITHDRAWAL—Kick It! Day 8, as needed.

I agree to rid my environment of tobacco, cigarettes, matches, lighters, ashtrays, and other smoking paraphernalia.

I am quitting smoking for myself, and of my own free will and I'm choosing to do so for the following reasons:

MY 5 MOST IMPORTANT BENEFITS OF QUITTING:

1. _____

2. _____

3. _____

4. _____

5. _____

Signed _____

Dated _____

PHASE 2: COLD TURKEY

KICK IT! DAY 9: HEALING AND LETTING GO

PLEASE CONTINUE TO SMOKING YOUR e-CIGARETTE — ZERO MG NICOTINE, FLAVOR ONLY FILTER

Reminder:

- Rid your environment of cigarettes, all forms of tobacco and all smoking paraphernalia — matches, lighters, ashtrays, etc.

HOMEWORK: PLEASE READ *NOW*

You now have all the tools to integrate into your healing process and Be The Cause of your new and evolved non-smoking life. Think of your transformation — inside and out:

- You are no longer chemically addicted to the drug nicotine;
- You now have a way of coping with the feelings you used to shove down with cigarettes;
- You've learned to turn off the love affair with your habit;
- And, most importantly... You have relapse prevention skills, understanding that one puff on a cigarette re-addicts!

CRUTCH VS. HEALTHY SUBSTITUTE

Your e-Cigarette is your smoking substitute — not a crutch.

A substitute is something you use until the original thing is no long needed. An unhealthy crutch is something different. The key: Distinguish between a want and a need. You may want to continue e-Smoking (nicotine free of course), and you may even need it while you adjust to stopping smoking, but if you find that you use them as a constant crutch, there's a good chance that you are using them to mask the feelings that you shoved down with smoking. This masking interrupts your emotional development and healing.

Enjoy your e-Cigarette, but don't let it be a substitute to avoid expressing feelings head on! As you know, when you stop smoking, you activate Panel 6 — Explosions.

When emotions suppressed by smoking resurface, they can create a war within and without (Panel 6). The only psychologically healthy way to deal with your emotions is to let them out — cry, rage, or grieve if you have to, and use your communication skills to make sure that you don't kill any relationships in the process. If and when you are ready, you can make a choice to Let Go of your e-Cigarette, or hold onto it for harmless fun.

THE SENSE THAT SOMETHING'S MISSING

If the dizziness, the light-headedness, the inability to concentrate and the constant craving for tobacco are beginning to fade, it's because the nicotine has left your bloodstream and you're no longer chemically addicted. If you're still experiencing symptoms of nicotine withdrawal, relax. Your body is just taking a little longer to rid itself of the drug.

Just because you may be through nicotine withdrawal doesn't necessarily mean that you're home free. After all the time you've spent as a smoker did you really expect your urges to disappear in a few short easy sessions? Let's be realistic. Adapting psychologically to not smoking is a step-by-step process. Each day gets easier and easier, but you still miss your cigarettes.

Why?

It's normal if:

- You have a feeling that something's missing in your life;
- You have a feeling of emptiness;
- You're at a loss for something to do or say.

The e-Cigarette and all the other substitutes you learned about in the past few days will help fill this void, but until you adjust to your new nonsmoking routine, the feeling that something's missing may persist until it eventually fades.

It will.

In the meantime, appreciate that your purse, pockets and life aren't cluttered up with cigarettes, lighters, matches and other smoking paraphernalia. In this case, something's missing — in a good way.

A SENSE OF LOSS

Sometimes a feeling of loss goes much deeper. Some ex-smokers — and you may be one of them — go through an intense and emotionally difficult time — a grieving process similar to losing a best friend. After all, cigarettes were always there for you to help take away your pain, and/ or keep you company during lonely times when you needed something to lean on.

Many ex-smokers have sat in my office crying. Yes, crying and grieving over the loss of their best friend, the cigarette.

Many ex-smokers, and you may be one of them, have been using cigarettes to fill that empty feeling I call the "hole in the soul." Sometimes cigarettes become emotional crutches that mask feelings of emptiness within, the origins of which date back to the bonding or lack thereof you received from your primary caretaker during the first 3 years of life. When the mother-baby bonding and attachment is inconsistent or insecure, the human need for connection is interfered with, leaving you with an inability to self sooth, setting you up for habits and addictions that serve the purpose of soothing you, but don't necessarily enhance your well-being. Quitting smoking can trigger old, and unconscious attachment breaks during early childhood development. These attachment breaks can be healed through grieving these wounds and morning the loss of unmet needs. Through self love and the love of and support of others, healing can take place.

6 STAGES OF GRIEF

Dr. Elizabeth Kübler-Ross researched death and the dying and found that those who have lost a loved one go through 6 Stages of Grief. Giving up cigarettes, for some, can feel like losing a loved one.

Here are the stages and how they apply to your sense of loss:

STAGE 1: ANGER – If you're feeling angry, it's because you're probably rebelling against your loss. It may sound like this: "I don't want to be uncomfortable! Give me back my pacifier." Even the most mature individuals find themselves regressing to this childlike state.

Talk empathically to yourself. You might say, "I know I'm angry, but I get even angrier thinking about how cigarettes controlled me for so many years. I'd rather be temporarily angry than permanently sick."

STAGE 2 AND 3: DENIAL AND BARGAINING – They go hand in hand. You got through smoking one day at a time by fooling yourself that quitting smoking is temporary (denial), in exchange for the bargain or deal — that you could smoke during your counter-conditioning exercises. Bargaining sounds like, "I can quit for 24 hours at a time. I'll even quit for another 24 hours if I can smoke again, tomorrow."

At some point deniers and bargainers have to face reality and resolve to a lifetime commitment. This doesn't mean that you should no longer quit smoking 24 hours at a time. You can still face the reality of quitting permanently while making day-by-day commitments.

STAGE 4: SADNESS — Because you are saying goodbye to something you looked at as a companion (even if that companion was doing you harm), it's one you've know intimately. Cry, grieve if you need to. It's part of your healing process.

Because you are using the e-Cigarette or oral substitute to replace your smoking habit, you may find that you may not be missing your cigarettes as much as you thought you would.

STAGE 5: DEPRESSION — At some point, you may have a deep realization that you have stopped smoking for good. It's an internal Letting Go (Panel 4) of all hope to ever smoke again. It's a point where you psychologically bottom out, and a necessary part of your process towards your last stage...

STAGE 6: ACCEPTANCE — This is where you no longer need to fight with yourself to continue the process you began. Acceptance is not a point you reach, but a process that you find yourself working towards. With acceptance comes relief and the knowledge that you are no longer under the spell of smoking.

So, though you may feel sad, angry, depressed and lost — remember these feelings are temporary...and normal.

KILLING THE 'TIL-DEATH-DO-US-PART' CONTRACT

Years ago, when you bought your first pack of cigarettes, you entered into a contract with the tobacco company. Without realizing it, you agreed to buy their product no matter what the cost. You continued to use this product in spite of its bad taste, bad smell and unhealthy effects.

Sometimes you chose it over your friends, your significant spouse/ significant other, or even your children. Many of you even chose heart disease, emphysema and cancer over quitting smoking. In short, you continued to honor your contract with the tobacco company no matter what the consequences.

How did the tobacco companies seduce more than 50 million Americans?

There are two answers:

The first is addiction (especially with the addition of free-base nicotine). The cigarette's magically addictive quality makes it a marketer's dream. What could be a more perfect product to sell than one with a little something contained within to make the buyer want more and more... all the time.

The second aspect to your 'Til-Death-Do-Us-Part' contract with the tobacco company is image. It's probably why you began smoking in the first place, why you endured the dizziness and the nausea of your first few cigarettes, and why you chose your particular brand.

To create an image that captivated you into making your contract with your particular brand, tobacco companies spend billions of dollars a year in marketing, advertising and package design.

You know the images I'm talking about:

Marlboro —The strongly independent, self-reliant "Marlboro Man." Smoke them and you too can feel rugged adventurous, and sexy.

Virginia Slims — The successful and sexy liberated woman. Smoke them and you will feel young, slim, and beautiful, at any age and at any weight!

Cool — Fresh, young, athletic, healthy, the outdoors! With this image in mind, you would think that smoking Cool is like being up in the mountains breathing fresh air!

The tobacco companies have worked hard to create these images, and they've been extremely successful. After all, they hooked you, didn't they?

Congratulations! You unhooked yourself from your habit and addiction. Take a few moments to unhook from the brainwashing.

Redo these ads in your mind's eye. Deconstruct the message and the manipulation.

See the Marlboro Man riding on his horse hooked to an oxygen machine.

See the Virginia Slims Girl smiling, showing off stained yellowed teeth, wrinkles and bloodshot eyes.

See yourself in the Cool Outdoors, coughing, wheezing, barely able to catch your breath and enjoy the fresh air.

Take a moment to remember what hooked you into your brand and deconstruct the image. Start your own anti-cigarette mental ad campaign. It costs you nothing but a little imagination, and it's part of the antidote to the manipulation you've been drawn into. The next time you see a smoking ad, use your imagination to rip the false message to shreds.

VISUALIZATION: JOURNEY THROUGH YOUR MIND MAP

"To" Healing and Freedom: Panels 7-9

You have arrived at LIGHT (Panel 7), and your final journey "To" Healing and Freedom.

Look at your Mind Map, Panel 7 and notice the interconnecting orbs generating LIGHT. As you continue to embark on your Visual Journey through Panels 7-9, acknowledge that your hard work generated the LIGHT that creates HEALING and FREEDOM. As you visually flow through the last row of Panels, remember:

You Caused the LIGHT — The shift from Addiction to Healing and Freedom!

Take a few minutes to see yourself flow through your Mind Map. You have traveled "From," "Through" and "To" Panels 7-9 — LIGHT, HEALING, AND FREEDOM.

Read this first before beginning your Visual Journey:

Step into Panel 7: LIGHT. Notice the light emanating from the center of the interconnected orbs. Step into the center of the LIGHT — your source of power to Be The Cause of the integration of your mind, body and Being.

Feel the warmth and comfort of the light, and watch it's power burn away old memories of you habit and addiction.

Step into Panel 8: HEALING. Immerse yourself in healing waters of the blue ocean and allow the DNA strands to envelop and heal you mentally and physically.

Step into Panel 9: FREEDOM. See yourself swimming freely in the ocean waters as you encounter the 3 Dolphins. The Dolphins are there to greet you and remind you of the 3 pieces of wisdom you earned along your Journey "From," "Through," "To."

> The first dolphin represents the wisdom you earned through your mind.

> The second dolphin represents the wisdom you earned through your body.

> The third dolphin represents the wisdom you earned through your Being.

You have earned the power to Be The Cause of your success.

You have arrived at your final destination and the beginning of your ongoing future success:

Congratulations ex-smoker! You've kicked the habit and addiction, permanently, a day-at-a-time!

The American Cancer Society lists the following benefits of quitting smoking:

20 minutes after quitting: Your heart rate and blood pressure drop.

2 hours after quitting: The carbon monoxide level in your blood drops to normal.

2 weeks to 3 months after quitting: Your circulation improves and your lung function increases.

1 to 9 months after quitting: Coughing and shortness of breath decrease; cilia (tiny hair like structures that move mucus out of the lungs) regain

normal function in the lungs, increasing the ability to handle mucus, clean the lungs and reduce the risk of infection.

1 year after quitting: The excess risk of coronary heart disease is half that of a smoker's.

2 to 5 years after quitting: Your stroke risk is reduced to that of a nonsmoker.

10 years after quitting: The lung cancer death rate is about half that of a person who continues smoking. The risk of cancer of the mouth, throat, esophagus, bladder, cervix and pancreas decrease.

15 years after quitting: The risk of coronary heart disease is the same as a nonsmoker's.

Information from the American Cancer Society.

IMPORTANT REMINDERS:

ONE THOUGHT RE-ADDICTS: NEVER FLIRT WITH YOUR DESIRE TO SMOKE! It's a mental trick that will sabotage you back to smoking. Instead, rewire your desire and kill it with your Sense Memory Technique. Practice it as many times as you have a craving.

ONE PUFF RE-ADDICTS: NEVER SMOKE BETWEEN SESSIONS! One puff on a cigarette (other than when instructed to do so in the exercises) will re-addict you by turning you back "on" to smoking!

Note: Use your Quitter's Survival Guide (refer to it often) for quick helpful reminders about quitting.

Keep the glass jar of water and cigarettes for at least another week to remind you of your filthy habit and addiction.

PLEASE SIGN YOUR DAY 9 (FINAL CONTRACT) AND RETURN TOMORROW AT YOUR SCHEDULED TIME.

PHASE 2: COLD TURKEY

HABIT BREAKERS COLD TURKEY

STOP SMOKING CONTRACT FOR KICK IT! DAY 9

MY FINAL CONTRACT

I _____, commit to quitting smoking cigarettes permanently.

I agree to follow the nicotine dosage schedule below:

- Kick It! Day 9 and Beyond: Continue smoking your e-Cigarette – Zero mg nicotine filter, flavor only for as long as you like. It's your choice. Be conscious about using it as a temporary cigarette substitute and not as a psychological crutch.

I understand and agree that I will not "cheat" and smoke cigarettes any time, or use nicotine replacement therapy (NRT — gums, patches, or any other form of nicotine, etc.) ever.

I agree to continue to live in a smoke free environment free from tobacco, cigarettes, matches, lighters, ashtrays, and other smoking paraphernalia.

I am quitting smoking for myself, and of my own free will and will continue to acknowledge my newfound health and freedom.

I hereby agree to exit out of the contract that I unconsciously signed up for with the tobacco company. The deal was more than I bargained for, and I'm no longer willing to pay the 'til death do us part' consequences I've incurred and would continue to incur by continuing to smoke.

I am hereby making a conscious decision to quit smoking permanently, one day at a time, and dissolve all the chains that shackled me to this habit and addiction.

If I should relapse and smoke again, I commit to getting back on track immediately, within less than 24 hours.

Signed (of my own free will) _____

Dated_____

PHASE 2: COLD TURKEY

KICK IT! DAY 10: STAYING QUIT

PLEASE CONTINUE SMOKING YOUR e-CIGARETTE – ZERO MG NICOTINE, FLAVOR ONLY FILTER

Reminder:

- Rid your environment of cigarettes, all forms of tobacco and all smoking paraphernalia — matches, lighters, ashtrays, etc.

HOMEWORK: PLEASE READ *NOW*

In this chapter you'll find 5 sections that will help you **stay quit permanently**! Re-read and use them whenever you have the urge to smoke or use food as a cigarette substitute.

HABIT BREAKERS HOTLINE

In 1978, UCLA established a crisis-intervention Stay-Quit hotline. It was a seven-day-a-week service set up to stop ex-smokers from relapsing. Before the ex-smoker would light up a cigarette, he or she would call to get help from a trained counselor ready to assist. In November of 1980, this federally-funded hotline ran out of money, but the project sparked an idea that proved a valuable tool for the Habit Breakers Stop Smoking Program.

When I opened the Habit Breakers Stop Smoking Clinic in 1980, I incorporated a 24-hour crisis intervention hotline to help prevent smokers from relapsing. Before enrolling, each client agreed to call the hotline before lighting a cigarette.

From my experience with handling hundreds of callers, I learned why ex-smokers relapse, and how best to counsel them through their urge to smoke. I'd like to share some relapse prevention conversations in the hopes that you can learn more relapse prevention skills.

THE UPSET WOMAN

A client called me months after quitting smoking. She was very agitated when she related the following incident:

Ex-smoker: My car was robbed. I just bought it the other day and it's gone. I'm so angry I could explode. I need to calm down. I need a cigarette.

Dr. Judy: You sound very upset. It would have been so easy to buy a pack of cigarettes rather than to place this call, but you didn't.

Ex-smoker: That's true. But I'd sure like to have a cigarette this minute.

Dr. Judy: It seems like your just want to get rid of your anger and then get on with life as an ex-smoker.

Ex-smoker: Yes

Dr. Judy: Amy you've been off cigarettes for 3 months now. You've successfully handled many stressful events in this time frame. What has kept you from smoking?

Ex-smoker: Knowing that lighting up won't make the situation better. I've worked too hard to quit smoking to start smoking again and re-addict myself.

Dr. Judy: OK, calm down, breathe through your nose, to the top of your head, and down your body. *Ground* the craving like grounding static electricity. Appreciate how clear and uncongested your chest feels and reaffirm your decision to remain quit. Do you remember why you chose to quit?

Ex-smoker: Yes. I want to be able to exercise better, and I want to be in control of my life and not have cigarettes control *me.*

Dr. Judy: Sounds to me like you're ready to get on with things and deal with this unfortunate incidence without smoking. Can you commit to not smoking for the next 24 hours?

Ex-smoker: Yes, absolutely.

Dr. Judy: Let's talk again tomorrow.

THE EXPLOSIVE EMPLOYEE

Ex-smoker: I can't stand working for my boss any longer. I want to tell him what I really think of him and then flatten his face against the wall.

Dr. Judy: And on top of that you can't even numb these feeling by sucking them down with a cigarette.

Ex-smoker: Exactly. It's not easy to resist reaching for a cigarette when I'm feeling this way. Sometimes I want to say "What the heck. Life's hard enough without trying to quit smoking too." I'm calling because I made a commitment to call you before lighting up a cigarette, and I want you to know that I have one in my hand now.

Dr. Judy: OK John. How is smoking going to make your life better?

Ex-smoker: Well, for one, it will keep me from saying or doing something I may regret later.

Dr. Judy: Are you afraid to feel this angry for fear of say something out of control and get fired for it?

Ex-smoker: That's right.

Dr. Judy: What's the worst thing that can happen from *feeling* this way?

Ex-smoker: I told you, I can lose control, punch the guy out, or say the wrong thing and get fired.

Dr. Judy: But you didn't, did you? You left the situation to make this phone call.

Ex-smoker: That's true.

Dr. Judy: John, there's a big difference between *feeling* and *acting*. If I acted on all my feelings, I'd be behind bars. Do you get the difference?

Ex-smoker: I got it. Just because I have a *feeling*, it doesn't mean that I have to *act* on it right?

Dr. Judy: Right. If you feel uncomfortable, leave the situation, and go back to resolve the problem after you've cooled off. Let's review the Sense Memory Technique before we hang up the phone.

Ex-smoker: Sure.

Dr. Judy: Imagine lighting up a cigarette. Picture yourself inhaling the heavy, sooty, bitter smoke. Feel your chest swell with congestion.... can you feel it?

Ex-smoker: Yes.

Dr. Judy: Now use your Sense Memory to bring back the dizziness, the irritability, and the nausea that you experienced in the course of your treatment.

Ex-smoker: OK, I've got it.

Dr. Judy: Imagine inhaling again... cough, hard. Again, *harder*. Can you agree not to smoke for the next 24 hours?

Ex-smoker: Yes (coughing). I'm fine.

Dr. Judy: How about destroying the cigarette in your hand and flushing it down the toilet?

Ex-smoker: Fine.

Dr. Judy: You kept your commitment. That is the source of your power. Call again if you need to.

THE CAGED ANIMAL

Ex-smoker: I feel like a caged animal. I keep pacing back and forth and I don't know how to calm down.

Dr. Judy: For eight years you've been calming yourself down with a cigarette. No wonder you feel this way.

Ex-smoker: I'm not sure I can do this.

Dr. Judy: This is only your first day without nicotine. Withdrawal makes it easy to forget the fact that you *chose* to quit smoking. The addiction plays a trick on you and makes it seem as though the idea was "imposed" by an outside force. Remember, you're not a caged animal. You're freer than you ever were because *you, not your cigarettes*, are calling the shots on your smoking habit. In a little while you'll be past this experience and feeling differently about things. In the mean time, let's go through a deep breathing exercise to help you relax.

Starting with a deep breath in through the nose, breath all the way up to the top of you head and exhale the stress of the day down your body, into the ground. Use your breath to soothe yourself. Do this a couple of times until you feel more grounded and less anxious. Can you commit to another 24 hours without smoking?

Ex-smoker: I'm not sure.

Dr. Judy: 12 hours?

Ex-smoker: Yes. I'm going to bed soon and I can't smoke while I sleep, fortunately.

Dr. Judy: Call back in the morning and let me know how you feel.

THE OBSESSIVE EX-SMOKER

Ex-smoker: I'm starting to obsess about smoking. I can't get cigarettes out of my mind. It's just a matter of time before I give into this nagging urge.

Dr. Judy: You sound like a walking time bomb ready to explode.

Ex-smoker: Right. I just want to get cigarettes off my mind, and the only way to stop obsessing about them is by giving in to them.

Dr. Judy: You lost another job and you want to smoke to numb the pain, right?

Ex-smoker: How did you guess?

Dr. Judy: What are you doing about getting another job?

Ex-smoker: Obsessing about cigarettes.

Dr. Judy: I see. Do you see how smoking makes you passive? How it keeps you from taking action and looking for another job? It's your Defense Mechanism (Panel 5). When you obsess about smoking, you don't have to face the pain, anger, shame and disappointment of being unemployed. Sheila, you already made the decision to quit smoking. It's *not negotiable*. There's clearly only one thing left to do.

Ex-smoker: What's that?

Dr. Judy: Keep your word to yourself! Do you want to see your urges disappear?

Ex-smoker: Yes.

Dr. Judy: Then put yourself on the line 100%. Re-Commit.

Ex-smoker: I guess I can do that . . .

Dr. Judy: *Guessing* isn't good enough. You have to put yourself on the line 100%.

Ex-smoker: It's a *no-win* situation. When I smoke, I want to quit. When I'm not smoking, I want to light up. Is there any *hope* for me?

Dr. Judy: No. *Hoping* to succeed doesn't work Sheila. Put yourself on the line with this. Choose to make an absolute commitment to quit smoking for the next 24 hours.

Ex-smoker: OK. I choose to make an absolute commitment for 24 hours.

Dr. Judy: Now watch your urge to smoke disappear. Remember: Urges feed on *hope* which then creates *obsessions*. If there's *no hope* for a cigarette, urges are of no value. Enjoy an un-obsessive day. I'll talk to you tomorrow.

WEIGHT CONTROL

Quitting smoking and gaining weight don't necessarily have to go together. Even though gaining weight is a big concern, only one third of those who quit smoking do so. It's because they substitute food for cigarettes and "abuse" food just as they "abused" cigarettes.

You can suck your feelings down with a cigarette, and you can swallow your feelings using food. You can attempt to reduce stress by smoking, and you can attempt to do it with food. You can pick your energy level up by smoking a stimulant — nicotine, or you can do it with sugar and eat a candy bar. Both substances peak your blood sugar level and give you a quick energy fix. It's too easy to switch from one stimulant (nicotine) to another (sugar).

Today you're going to apply some of the same techniques you learned to handle your urge to smoking, to your urge to overeat and prevent yourself from gaining weight — another way to sabotage your success.

The obvious difference between giving up smoking and giving of overeating is that you can go Cold Turkey on cigarettes, but you can't with food — nor would you want to. But what you *can* do is stop the attitudes, behaviors, and bad food choices that create excess weight gain.

Let's take a look at what you can do to gain control of overeating.

RULE 1: DON'T DIET

If you want to lose weight and keep it off, you have to give up dieting. ___Dieting doesn't work___ because you can't stay on a diet for the rest of your life. The mind remembers everything you wanted to eat when you were on a diet, and reminds you to eat everything you were so successful at avoiding.

The resultant effect is the **yo-yo syndrome**. You go on a diet. Your weight comes off. You feel deprived. You eat. You gain it all back again. Then you start the cycle all over again.

RULE 2: MAKE EVERY MEAL COUNT

What works is the _opposite_ depriving yourself. **Make every meal special** — an orally and sensually satisfying experience. You can do that without eating fattening foods and gaining excess weight. It simply takes a little imagination and effort:

- Create "atmosphere" when you sit down for a meal. Make your table beautiful — flowers, colorful setting, candles, music, etc. Drink from a wine glass filled with club soda or mineral water with lemon or lime.

- Eat foods that you love, chosen from healthy food groups. Use herbs and spices (instead of salt) to kick up some flavor.

- Include desserts. Don't deprive yourself. Satisfy your need for dessert by eating healthy ones — fruit, low fat yogurt, ice cream (sugar free), even home-prepared desserts (use whole wheat flour, stevia, Truvia or agave for a sweetener). Be creative!

- Now that your sense of taste and smell is better than ever, you can enjoy the subtle taste of good food, and need less sugar and salt. Win/win!

RULE 3: EAT SLOWLY

When you sit down to eat, make it a time to relax. Put on your favorite music, turn off the phone and enjoy your meal.

Eating slowly is key to losing weight. It takes 20 minutes for the brain to get the message that you're full, so slow down and make your meal last at last 20 minutes. To help you slow down:

- Put your fork and knife down between bites;
- Chew slowly and enjoy every morsel of food;
- Drink water between bites;
- Breathe deeply and frequently to avoid wolfing down a meal and overeating.

RULE 4: USE ORAL SUBSTITUTES

Most of the time what you have in your mouth is not as important as having something to keep it busy with. Popcorn (nonfat), rice cakes, celery, carrots, green peppers, sunflower seeds (watch the quantity because they are high in calories) sugarless gum/mints, a straw, a coffee stirrer, toothpick, or even a cinnamon stick can satisfy your oral needs.

Remember: do not to get in the habit of substituting food for smoking!

If you have the urge to eat, drink a glass of water or some herbal tea before reaching for food. You may find that your urge will go away. Brush your teeth or gargle with mouthwash. You'll think twice about eating when your breath tastes sweet and clean.

It's a good idea to get in the habit of brushing your teeth right after eating. Make it a ritual.

RULE 5: DON'T SKIP OR SKIMP ON MEALS

If you want to control your weight, you want to make sure that you are eating well. It may sound counterintuitive, but it's not.

If you skip or eat small meals, you'll feel hungry between meals and have a tendency to either snack or overeat.

Eat five or six small meals throughout the day to keep your metabolism high and prevent your body from storing fat. Start with a high-protein breakfast, a mid morning snack, a medium sized lunch, an afternoon snack, and a light nutritious dinner, like a salad and roasted veggies, with some protein like tofu, chicken or fish. If you crave a certain dessert, remember not to deprive yourself. Just eat less of it.

RULE 6: PORTION CONTROL — THE KEY TO WEIGHT LOSS

Learn these 5 easy ways to keep your portion size correct:

- Rid your home of fattening foods — out of sight is out of mind;
- Serve your portions from the stove, not the table – it's a deterrent to spooning out extra portions;
- Don't eat everything on your plate – leave some leftovers;
- When dining out, order a la carte. Order more if you're still hungry;
- Ask the waiter to forego the bread and butter;
- Split a meal with a friend;
- Doggie bag. More to enjoy later.

RULE 7: EAT ONLY AT THE DINING TABLE

Eat only at the table and don't mix it with other activities such as reading or watching TV. It's easy to get carried away with the plot of a good book or TV show and unconsciously overeat.

RULE 8: TURN ON TO "THIN" FOODS. TURN OFF TO "FAT" FOODS

Just as you were able to use your Sense Memory to "turn off" to smoking, you can use it to "turn on" to healthy food.

SENSE MEMORY TECHNIQUE FOR FOOD:

Imagine that you've just eaten a fresh, light, nutritious salad. Taste the subtle flavors of the vegetables. Smell the fine aroma of herbs and spices. Experience how satisfied and good you feel afterwards.

Now imagine that you just polished off your favorite junk food. You feel stuffed, greasy, bloated and cramped.

Practice going back and forth between the Sense Memory of eating a nutritiously satisfying meal and overstuffing yourself on junk until the first starts feeling better.

It takes about 21 days to form good eating habits. Within a short time, these habits will be ingrained into your lifestyle.

Take these steps towards behavioral change one day at a time and prove to yourself that you can quit smoking and keep your weight under control!

PREVENTING RELAPSE: EIGHT COMMON TRAPS FOR FAILURE

It's relatively easy to stop smoking. The challenge is staying off permanently! To prevent yourself from relapsing and having to go Through the process of stopping smoking ever again, let's look at eight common traps for failure:

- Life crisis — death of a loved one, sickness, or divorce
- Drinking alcohol and abusing drugs (prescription or illegal)
- Eating with smokers
- Relaxing after dinner
- Pressure or frustration at work
- Arguments
- Depression
- Boredom

Since re-addiction could be triggered by one of the above situations, you want to be prepared to handle these common traps for failure. As you read the two scenarios below, imagine that you are in these situations and think about how you would behave under the circumstances.

DRINKING SCENARIO

It's after work. You were just promoted and the gang decides to take you out for a drink to celebrate. It occurs to you that you shouldn't be drinking so soon after you quit smoking, but you figure "How often do I get promoted?" You order just one glass of wine to "play it safe."

You start to loosen up and order another round of drinks. The cigarette in the ashtray next to you is looking better and better. See yourself reach for the cigarette in the ashtray...

STOP! GET YOUR FINGERS AWAY FROM THAT CIGARETTE!

Take a deep breath and flood your senses with negative Sense Memories – the bitter harsh taste, the feeling of nausea, the congestion and irritation in you chest. Cough, clear your throat, and get out of there! Go to the bathroom, splash some cold water on your face, brush your teeth, take a few deep breaths and go home — sober.

Let's go over these coping skills again: You're just about to pick up a cigarette...

> STOP!
>
> RECALL YOUR "TURN OFF" FEELINGS ABOUT SMOKING
>
> WASH YOUR FACE, BRUSH YOUR TEETH
>
> TAKE A DEEP BREATH
>
> LEAVE!

The more you practice this exercise, the more automatic your response to a similar situation will be. When you're drunk and vulnerable, you don't want to be planning prevention skills. Have your strategy planned out beforehand.

What's wrong with the about scenario? The answer is obvious. You shouldn't have been out drinking after quitting smoking in the first place!

Stay away from alcohol and any other drugs that interfere with your decision-making abilities for as long as possible. If you insist on drinking alcohol, make sure that there are no cigarettes around.

ARGUMENT SCENARIO

You've just had a major argument with your spouse or lover. Remember how cigarettes soothed your nerves when you were angry, how they helped smooth over your relationship problems?

Before you say or do something that you may regret later, you run out of the house, shaking with anger and drive to the store. There, sitting on the shelf, is your relief. You're just about to rip open the pack of cigarettes...

STOP! TEAR THAT PACKAGE TO SHREDS AND TRASH IT!

Even better, return it for a refund, and buy yourself something else instead. How about sugarless gum or a magazine?

Go through this scene again, carefully thinking through what you could do instead of going to the store to buy a pack of cigarettes.

Other options? How about cooling off emotionally before acting impulsively? Take a shower — you can't smoke in the shower. Jog and run off the tension. Punch a pillow.

When you've cooled off, take a direct approach to handling what's bothering you. Get off your chest what you've been sucking down with a cigarette. Communicate with you partner directly without blaming, criticizing, judging, moralizing or yelling. Direct, effective communication is the best relief possible — even better than smoking. When you do so, you may find that the urge to smoke disappears.

When you take the time to rehearse in advance your traps for failure, you will continue to stay conscious of the addict within and outwit it at it's own sabotaging game. Be The Cause of your continued success and take the advice of a genius:

"Smart people solve problems. Geniuses prevent them." Albert Einstein

YOU ARE OFFICIALLY DONE WITH YOUR WITH YOUR STOP SMOKING PLAN.

PRINT and FRAME your GRADUATION CERTIFICATE to acknowledge your success.

Go to www.drjudyshabitbreakers.com to download a full colored version of your Graduation Certificate.

CONGRATULATIONS, EX-SMOKER!

PLEASE TAKE A MOMENT TO PRINT OUT YOUR GRADUATION CERTIFICATE

HABIT BREAKERS STOP SMOKING

GRADUATION CERTIFICATE

I, _____ hereby acknowledge that I have successfully completed the Habit Breakers Stop Smoking Plan on this day of _____ .

This is an acknowledgment of the completion of my journey *FROM ADDICTION, TO FREEDOM*, and the commencement of my smoke-free life.

Congratulations On Your Accomplishment to Breaking the Habit and Addiction of Smoking

Wishing You the Best of Health,

Judy Rosenberg, Ph. D.

Judy Rosenberg, Ph.D.

JUDY

IN CASE OF RELAPSE

SUPPLIES:

ONE PACK OF YOUR LEAST FAVORITE BRAND OF CIGARETTES (DON'T BUY THEM UNTIL RIGHT BEFORE YOUR SESSION, AND DON'T OPEN THE PACK UNTIL YOU ARE INSTRUCTED TO DO SO), GLASS JAR WITH WATER, LIGHTER OR MATCHES.

If you've been smoking for more than one day, repeat Days 6-8 (first 3 days of your counter-conditioning exercises), to successfully quit smoking again. If you've been smoking for less tha24 hours, do the exercise in this section.

If you feel guilty or embarrassed that you've let yourself down, remember that It takes a lot of integrity to keep your word and get back on track. The fact that you're reading this is proof that you want to quit again. And you will. Starting now.

Let's leave guilt, shame, and feeling like a failure on the sidelines. They are Defense Mechanisms designed to sabotage your attempt to quit smoking. These Defense Mechanisms lower your self-esteem and prevent you from getting back on track.

The good news is that if you've smoked only a few cigarettes, you aren't totally chemically re-addicted. You get a break from having to go through nicotine withdrawal all over again. The bad news is that you are psychologically re-addicted, and you probably found out the hard way that one puff on a cigarette will indeed re-addict.

As a matter of fact, by smoking again, you've wiped out all the negative associations you've worked so hard to establish in your counter-conditioning sessions. To help you re-establish them, you are going to do some more "turn off" style smoking today.

But first, take a few minutes to recall your 5 most important consequences of smoking and benefits of quitting:

CONSEQUENCES OF SMOKING:

- _____
- _____
- _____
- _____
- _____

BENEFITS OF QUITTING:

- _____
- _____
- _____
- _____
- _____

COUNTER-CONDITIONING EXERCISE:

As you go through the exercise, keep these reasons in the forefront of your mind.

Ready? Open your pack of cigarettes. Light up.

1. Inhale -- suck it down deep -- cough, hard.

2. Inhale -- cough again, harder.

3. Inhale – cough -- feel the bitterness on your lips and tongue.

4. Inhale -- cough,-- feel the heat and congestion in your chest.

5. Inhale – cough -- feel the irritation in your throat.

6. Inhale -- cough -- feel the heaviness in your chest.

7. Inhale -- cough -- feel the stinging in your eyes.

8. Inhale -- cough -- taste the staleness in your mouth.

9. Inhale – cough -- say goodbye to your last cigarette.

10. Inhale on your e-Cigarette and feel the difference.

If you still have a strong urge to smoke, repeat this exercise. Stop if you feel sick. When you're ready, throw your cigarette butts and your unused cigarettes into the jar of water.

Wash up, brush your teeth, drink some cold water, and RETURN back here when you're done.

RELAPSE ANALYSIS

Let's take a moment to study the situation that caused you to relapse.

How soon after the relapse are you reading this and getting back on track?_____

How long were you off cigarettes before you relapsed?_____

When did you relapse?_____

How soon did you need another cigarette after you relapsed?_____

How much have you been smoking daily since the relapse?_____

Where were you when you relapsed?_____

Who were you with?_____

What was the feeling that triggered the relapse?_____

Judy Rosenberg, Ph.D.

What was the environment that triggered the relapse?_____

How did you feel after you lit up?_____

How did the first puff on your cigarette taste?_____

Why are you deciding to quit again?_____

Look over the above and ask yourself what you would do differently in the trigger situation.

It is important to get back on track immediately. Once you start smoking, it's very difficult to break away from the habit and addiction and even more difficult to remember why you chose to quit in the first place.

IMPORTANT REMINDERS:

ONE THOUGHT RE-ADDICTS: NEVER FLIRT WITH YOUR DESIRE TO SMOKE! It's a mental trick that will sabotage you back to smoking. Instead, rewire your desire and kill it with your Sense Memory Technique. Practice it as many times as you have a craving.

ONE PUFF RE-ADDICTS: NEVER SMOKE BETWEEN SESSIONS! One puff on a cigarette (other than when instructed to do so in the exercises) will re-addict you by turning you back "on" to smoking!

Note: Use your Quitter's Survival Guide (refer to it often) for quick helpful reminders about quitting.

Take a moment to sign a contract with yourself and renew your commitment to quitting smoking.

HABIT BREAKERS STOP SMOKING

COMMITMENT RENEWAL CONTRACT

I,_____
_____, commit to quitting smoking for the next 24 hours, and will continue to quit smoking a day-at-a-time.

I've rid my environment of cigarettes, and all other smoking paraphernalia. I will not purchase any more tobacco products — EVER.

I will use the techniques I've learned in this last session to cope with the next 24 hours without a cigarette and will continue to use the techniques I've learned in my Plan to stay quit permanently.

In the event of relapse, I commit to getting back on track IMMEDIATELY!

I am quitting smoking for myself, and of my own free will and I'm choosing to do so for the following reasons:

BENEFITS OF QUITTING: Choose 5 most important reasons for quitting:

1. _____

2. _____

3. _____

4. _____

5. _____

Signed _____

Dated _____

QUITTER'S SURVIVAL GUIDE

(reference often)

A little friendly support to help you survive quitting smoking <u>one day at a time</u>.

- Breathe frequently through the day — inhale and imagine breath flowing from the top of your head into the ground.
- Find a focal point, focus, and breathe as you push the urge further and further into space.
- Use your tobacco-free e-Cigarette as a smoking substitute.
- Use your Sense Memory to "turn off" to smoking.
- Use your Fantasy Smoking technique to "turn on" to the fresh clean feeling of breathing.
- Use your oral and tactile substitutes to fill in the void.
- Make a crisis intervention call and talk your way through your urge.
- Take a whiff of the smoked butts in your jar.
- Review your reasons for quitting smoking.
- Don't flirt with your desire to smoke, EVER!

OTHER IMPORTANT SUGGESTIONS:

- Eat fresh organic foods — lots of fruits, vegetables, and whole grains.
- Don't skip meals.
- Supplement your diet with the vitamins and minerals throughout and after quitting smoking.
- Drink at least 6 to 8 glasses of water a day.
- Exercise and stretch frequently — sweat out the toxins.

- Take frequent hot baths, saunas or Jacuzzi — relax and unwind.

- Stop smoking a-day-at-a-time.

REMEMBER:

<u>ONE THOUGHT RE-ADDICTS</u>! NEVER FLIRT WITH YOUR DESIRE TO SMOKE!

<u>ONE PUFF READDICTS!</u> NEVER HAVE ANOTHER PUFF OFF A CIGARETTE AGAIN!

Contact Dr. Judy Rosenberg Ph.D.

If you have questions or concerns or would like to meet with Dr. Rosenberg on a personal basis you can contact Dr. Rosenberg via her website or call her office.

Dr. Judy's Habit Breakers Website: www.drjudyshabitbreakers.com or www.esmoke2quit.com

Dr. Judy's General Website:

www.drjudyrosenberg.com

Office: (818) 385-1815